Everything I Know About
Nutrition
I Learned from
BARLEY

Betty Kamen's Guide to Nutraceuticals and Functional Foods

Betty Kamen, PhD
and
Paul Kamen

Nutrition Encounter, Novato, California
www.bettykamen.com

All of the facts in this book have been very carefully researched from the scientific literature. In no way, however, are any of the suggestions meant to take the place of advice given by physicians. Please consult a medical or health professional should the need for one be indicated.

2002

Nutrition Encounter
PO Box 5847
Novato, CA 94948-5847
(415) 883-5154

Website: www.bettykamen.com

Email: betty@well.com

Printed in the United States of America
First Printing 2002

ISBN 0-944501-15-X

DEDICATED

to

Serafina Corsello, MD

~ who so willingly and graciously shares her genius for understanding the complexities of human biochemistry — a gift she skillfully uses to help everyone obtain optimum health

~ who dares to use techniques that don't fit accepted concepts, demonstrating how effective and safe they are

~ who helped me pry open nature's own healing secrets, especially those found in very particular green leaves

CONTENTS

DEDICATION   3

INTRODUCTION   6

CHAPTERS
1   A PLATE OF PREVENTION   14

2   BEYOND VITAMINS: THE NEXT   26
     LEVEL OF SUPPLEMENTATION

3   OUCH! YOU CUT YOUR FINGER   40

4   MY MOTHER, THE LATE-   52
     BLOOMING NUTRITION GURU

5   THE POWER OF GREEN   70

6   KNOW YOUR NUTRIENTS   86

7   MORE NUTRACEUTICALS   112
     AND FUNCTIONAL FOODS

8   WE *CAN* CONCENTRATE   134
     NATURE

9   GRAINS AS VEGETABLES   148
     OR GRAINS AS DRUGS?

ONE LINE. ONLINE DAILY   153
NUTRITION HINTS

ABOUT BETTY KAMEN   154

ABOUT PAUL KAMEN   155

ALSO FROM BETTY KAMEN   156

REFERENCES   158

INDEX   165

Editing
David Hennessy

~ ~ ~

Cover Design
Raylene Buehler

INTRODUCTION

...in which we tell the story of just how and when our modern-day nutritional status began to decline, long long ago.

Our story begins with a young woman who lived about 10,000 years ago. We don't know exactly where she lived, who she was, or what she looked like. But we think we know what she did, and we know all too well about the profound changes in the way people live and eat today as a result of her efforts.

Ten thousand and two years ago, in the summer of 8,000 BC, this woman settled into her chores for the day. First, she finished weaving a large basket for collecting wheat grains, a basket that balanced comfortably on her head.

As she worked, several of the younger children drew close while she told them a story she had heard when she herself was little – about a time in the distant past when their clan hunted for food. It was before the earth deities had shown their ancestors how to grow wheat and barley, and gave them the steady and reliable food supply that allowed them to settle into a permanent village.

"In those ancient days," she explained, "there were no fields of wheat, and no tilling, planting, watering, harvesting, and milling. We wandered the earth in search of good hunting."

Although the standard wisdom of her time was that agriculture was a gift from the gods, this particular young woman had to wonder if travel and hunting might not have been a much more exciting lifestyle than the tedious hours she spent in the field and over the milling stones.

"Does that mean that Grandfather didn't have wheat-meal mush and grain cakes?" asked a little boy.

"Grandfather had everything we have," she answered, "but his grandfather's grandfather only ate wheat and barley as they grew in the wild. In those days they ate the young sprouts as sweet vegetables, the grain kernels were tasty snacks along the trail."

Later that day, when this woman was working near the boundary between two different fields of grain, she noticed something strange: A few of the plants bore unusually large kernels. One of the fields had been planted with einkorn wheat, a now all-but-forgotten ancient variety. The other field was planted with emmer or Persian wheat, a grain that produces slightly larger kernels, although somewhat more difficult to cultivate. It was typical in those days for farmers to plant several varieties as a hedge against adverse weather or pest damage.

Our ancient farmer noticed the scattering of these few different stalks, heavy with much bigger kernels than those growing in the cultivated fields. She recalled seeing these before; they appeared with regularity on the boundaries between the two fields. But she had never had any success getting the seeds to germinate past the second generation.

On that day, however, she had an idea. Those big kernels were just too tempting, and she was determined to try and grow them herself. She collected some of the hybrid kernels and planted them – on a hunch – near some kernels from other hybrids that she had gathered.

"Maybe one combination isn't enough," she reasoned. "If I can get combinations of combinations, then I'll have more different kinds of combinations, and perhaps the resulting seeds will be fertile enough to eventually plant an entire new field of these bigger kernels."

Her work went on for several growing seasons. With each new set of hybrids, she coaxed a few more of the seeds to germinate. She endured the ridicule of the skeptics in the clan, paying no attention to their scoffing.

Finally, she achieved some measure of success: At last, the new line of wheat could perpetuate itself, but not without continuing human intervention.

> As long as there were people around to plant the seeds, keep the einkorn and Persian varieties off the field, and scare the birds away, the yield of this new kind of wheat was considerably enhanced because of the oversized kernels.

Our hypothetical farmer, even though she was only thinking of feeding her family with a bigger harvest next year, has fired the starting gun for western civilization.

What was really going on at the edges of those fields?

Time for a short lesson in botany:

Wheat, like barley, rice, corn, rye, oats, and millet, is a member of the grass family. Different types of wheat are classified depending on how many chromosomes they contain in each cell. What are chromosomes? Microscopic rod-shaped structures inside the nucleus of every living cell. The chromosomes contain the genes, the DNA with the genetic information of the organism. Every cell of every individual of the same species has the same characteristic number of chromosomes. People, for example, have 46 chromosomes in each cell, arranged in 23 pairs. Gorillas have 48, cats have 38, hamsters have 22, fruit flies have 8.

Plants with extra copies of each chromosome pair are often characterized by "polyploid gigantism," bearing extra-large fruit or kernels. (Plants may be selectively bred that way, in an effort to end up with a new species with higher growth potential.)

Chromosomes usually come in pairs - that's what makes it possible for a cell to maintain all its genetic information when it divides into two new cells. The most ancient species of cereal grasses have 7 pairs of chromosomes, for a total of 14. These are also called diploid grasses, with two of each of chromsome.

Diploid wheat is still found wild, and is seldom cultivated. Einkorn wheat is also one of this group – an ancient variety, all but forgotten to modern agriculture. Barley, with a few exceptions, is also a diploid grain.

Tetraploid wheat species, with four chromosome sets (for a total of 28), are found growing wild but have also been cultivated extensively for thousands of years. These include emmer, durum, Persian, kamut, and poulard wheat. Some of these names may be familiar to those of you who have been interested in alternatives to common wheat.

The hexaploid group, with six sets of seven chromosomes for a total of 42, has a mysterious history. It appeared suddenly around 8,000 BC, and is very likely the result of deliberate crossing of two other types of grain – one from the diploid family and one from the tetraploid.

This is where we imagine our anonymous farmer had an important role to play.

That courageous and persevering woman could have been the first successful genetic engineer. The cultivation of wheat with those two extra sets of chromosomes – the hexaploid – is thought to have played a major role in the viability of many ancient civilizations. Our modern common wheat is a hexaploid. So are club wheat, spelt, shot, macha, and valvilovii.

Our farmer inadvertently started the human species on what some may regard as a long downhill slide, nutrition-wise.

Why a downhill slide? Because modern wheat has been modified to such an extent that tens of millions of people in North America alone are allergic to it! The closer an agricultural product is to its naturally evolved beginnings, the less likely it is to cause an allergic response. So it is not surprising to find that many people who are allergic to products made from modern wheat grains are much less sensitive to foods made with more ancient types of grains – barley, for example.

This is yet another demonstration showing us that nature knows better than science, or better than human interference. High yield, resistance to pests and disease, suitability for mechanized harvesting and milling, even color for pasta manufacturing, are among the selection criteria. These attributes do not contribute to nutritional content, a factor that is rarely considered.

Pest resistance may have a particularly strong relation to allergic response. A pest-resistant plant is not simply a better and stronger plant. The resistance comes from higher levels of the plant's own natural pesticides. In some cases, our allergic response is a reaction to these natural poisons.

It makes perfect sense that ancient, unmodified species are less likely to trigger allergies.

What are the other long-term health effects of this biochemical brew that has completely bypassed the natural selection process? We can only guess.

Barley is an important food because it winds the clock back to a time when grains had not yet been genetically modified by cross-breeding and selection. As cultivated now, barley is genetically similar to the naturally occurring wild plant. This is in sharp contrast to modern varieties of wheat, which, as we have seen, have been selected and crossbred for thousands of years to meet short-term nutritional goals. These include:

> bigger kernels
> more calories
> easier harvesting
> easier milling
> resistance to poor growing conditions
> plant-produced pesticides for insect resistance

Used as a vegetable instead of a grain, barley can help bring us back even further in time, when we ate only fresh-picked plants and fresh-caught game.

Nature is abundant with animal species that thrive on newly sprouted grasses. But no animals have evolved to thrive on the part of the plant that modern humans choose to eat.

Our story is not over. Perhaps it is a good thing for the reputation of that pioneering farmer that her name was lost to history. We imagine that some of the narrow-minded men of the clan – probably the same ones who ridiculed her during her years of apparent failure – were the ones who took credit for the discovery.

Meanwhile, as the new high-yield varieties she had developed became the dominant crop, our heroine had the good sense to recognize in her later years that her hybrid grains were nutritionally inferior to the more natural varieties. She knew that interfering with nature's design was not good.

She herself lived to be a great-grandmother – rare in those days – and was well known to her friends, family and acquaintances in all the surrounding villages as the cranky old woman with the strange ideas about health.

She even lost interest in making the pasta-like wheat meal or barley meal that were the staple foods of her time (a time before bread-baking became common). Instead, she was experimenting with the dried leaves of young barley sprouts, pounded into a paste and then sun-dried for storage, to be mixed with water and served to her reluctant family throughout the winter.

She noticed that these tiny blades of grass – loaded with as yet unidentified chlorophyll and densely packed with as yet unnamed antioxidant vitamins and enzymes – provided the needed energy boost for the day's activities, whether for the women tending to the children or the fields, or for the men and boys on their adventurous expeditions.

She knew that when the great herds of the plains survived the dry season or winter, nature provided them with the young, green sprouting grasses. This was the only vegetation many herbivores ate. It supplied their sole nutritional support from birth to old age. (And still does!)

Empirical evidence also taught her that when these grasses were harvested at a young age, they appeared to be more effective. It seemed obvious to her that we were not designed for agriculture; we were designed to eat what grows naturally, as well as what we can pick or catch.

She accepted the wisdom of the ages:

> **Green has always been associated with the health and vitality of all living things, including people.**

But she didn't know how to make these young leaves taste good, and when she finally died – too old for anyone to remember when she was born – the world's first nutraceutical went with her as her great-great-grandchildren breathed a sigh of relief.

Ten thousand years later, we think we may have finally caught up with that ancient nutritionist. *

At long last, nutraceuticals and functional foods are being recognized as the only way to reconcile our destructive food environment with the fundamental requirements of the human body.

And, perhaps most important of all, we have solved the problem of making young green barley sprouts in supplemental form taste good.

*Any similarity between that ancient nutrition lady and Betty Kamen is purely intentional.

CHAPTER ONE
A PLATE OF PREVENTION

..in which we discuss prevention through diet, explore the reasons why we don't eat our vegetables, discuss my own personal health journey, and summarize what this book is all about.

"The majority of cancers could be prevented through changes in diet and lifestyle. In the past it was thought that cancer developed solely because of genetic predisposition, but we now know that's probably not true."

The brazen sword of the American Medical Association came down hard when nutrition advocates (like me) uttered such statements only two or three decades ago. But this announcement was received with absolutely no dissension at an important meeting recently held in Washington, DC.

The topic was "The Potential of Phytochemicals in Food for Preventing Cancer." Dr. David Heber, director of the Center for Human Nutrition at the Los Angeles School of Medicine, added: "To delay cancer might really take years of a healthful, mostly plant-based diet."[1]

Current medical journals are replete with research confirming that whole foods – especially vegetables – can ward off degenerative disease and extend our lifespan.

Look at what modern medical journals are reporting about these many common health concerns:

Aging
Phytochemicals present in blueberries, spinach, and strawberries (which are antioxidant-rich foods) may also be beneficial in reversing the course of neuronal and behavioral aging. (*Journal of Neuroscience*[2])

Arthritis
Pigments that give foods their color can cut disease risk, and also ease the pain of arthritis. (*Newsweek*[3])

Asthma
Adolescents raised on farms have less asthma and allergy than their urban peers. Farm children eat more freshly picked, unprocessed whole foods than suburban or city children, among other major lifestyle differences. (*American Journal of Critical Care Medicine,*[4] *Journal of Asthma*[5])

Alzheimer's Disease
Data from an observational study of 5,395 people suggest that a diet high in antioxidants may reduce the risk of developing Alzheimer's disease. Volunteers who consumed the highest levels of antioxidants "appeared to reduce their risk of Alzheimer's disease by about 25 percent." (World Alzheimer Congress[6])

Bladder Cancer
A high intake of cruciferous vegetables may reduce the risk of bladder cancer in men. "Intake of cruciferous vegetables is inversely associated with bladder cancer risk," report the researchers. The rate of bladder cancer in men is three to four times higher than in women. (*Journal of the National Cancer Institute*[7])

Breast Cancer
High consumption of vegetables and related micronutrients exert a protective effect on breast cancer risk. However, the experts conclude that there is no statistical significance with the consumption of fruit. (*European Journal of Cancer*[8])

Cardiovascular Disease
The consumption of large amounts of walnuts appears to be associated with increased levels of two protective substances against cardiovascular morbidity. (*Preventive Medicine*[9])

Cataracts
Broccoli and spinach are most consistently associated with a lower risk of cataracts. (*American Journal of Clinical Nutrition*[10])

Cholesterol
A mixed green vegetable and fruit beverage decreases the level of low-density lipoprotein cholesterol (the negative kind) in people whose levels are dangerously high. (*Journal of Agriculture and Food Chemistry*[11])

Colon Cancer
To reduce the risk of colon cancer, dietary fiber is required from all sources, including five to seven servings of vegetables and fruits per day, as well as generous portions of whole-grain cereals. (*Gastroenterology,*[12] *American Journal of Clinical Nutrition*[13])

Diabetes
Frequent salad vegetable consumption is associated with a reduction in the risk of diabetes. (*Nahrung,*[14] *Journal of Clinical Epidemiology*[15])

Digestive Tract Cancer
The consumption of even small amounts of fish can protect against the risk of several cancers, especially of the digestive tract. (*American Journal of Clinical Nutrition*[16])

Diverticulosis
This disease is associated with a past frequency of meat consumption. There is no such correlation with the frequency of vegetable or fruit consumption. (*Diseases of the Colon and Rectum*[17])

Endometrial Cancer
The consumption of vegetables reduces the risk of endometrial cancer. (*Journal of the Moffit Cancer Center*[18])

Lung Function & Lung Cancer
Middle-aged men with above-average intakes of fruit and vegetables have better lung function than those with low intakes. Higher fruit and vegetable intakes were also associated with lower risks of lung cancer in women, and were protective in both men and women who had never smoked cigarettes. (*Thorax,*[19] *Journal of the National Cancer Institute*[20])

Osteoporosis
Studies confirm that the best way to prevent osteoporosis is to eat your vegetables. Bone mass could be increased with vegetable intake even in those women who have had hysterectomies. (*American Journal of Clinical Nutrition,*[21] *Nature*[22])

Prostate Cancer
Vegetable intake substantially lowers the risk of prostate cancer. Men who eat three or more servings of cruciferous vegetables (broccoli and cabbage) a week have a 41 percent decreased risk of developing prostate cancer, compared with those who eat less than one serving per week. (*Journal of the National Cancer Institute*[23])

Rheumatoid Arthritis
Consumption of cooked vegetables is associated with a decreased risk of rheumatoid arthritis. (*American Journal of Clinical Nutrition*[24])

Stroke
Eating four or more servings of fruits and vegetables a day may reduce the risk of stroke, according to a study published in the *American Journal of Clinical Nutrition.* (CBS Health Watch[25])

I don't know about you, but every time I see a compilation of research results like these I run to the kitchen in a frantic search for anything that's green and edible. And this is only a very small sample of the published research. Compare with isolated vitamin supplements: Often effective, but not nearly as consistent or compelling. It is evident that synergistic ingredients found in whole foods are essential for the action of a single nutrient.

Keep in mind that although fruits are frequently coupled with vegetables in health-promoting statements, many fruits do not confer the attributes offered by vegetables. An age-old formula dictates that for every fruit you eat, you should consume three portions of vegetables to balance the high carbohydrate content of the fruit. (Sorry about that!)

WHY WE DON'T EAT OUR VEGETABLES

"Your health will suffer because you are overweight, you eat too much junk food, and you don't get enough exercise."

These words (hopefully delivered a little more tactfully) have not initiated lifestyle changes for the majority of us, no matter how many times we have heard them. Information about the amazing health benefits of vegetables is common knowledge nowadays, but still most American dinner plates are sorely lacking in these essential nutrients. There are several pressing questions we must ask ourselves:

~ Why aren't we more willing to change our ways in light of the grim statistics of our health status?

~ Why the huge rift between what we know (or what we are told) and how we actually eat?

~ Why are death rates for our killer afflictions rising rapidly in a time that has been termed, ironically, the era of "health and awareness"?[26]

~ Why are Americans consuming the same high percentage of calories from energy-dense, nutrient-poor foods as they did in the 1970s, despite the explosion of information about health and diet?

It is natural to resist recommendations that are difficult to implement!

~ The flight attendant, even in first class, pays no attention to my request for a complex carbohydrate meal.
~ My friends do not serve more than one recognizable vegetable (if that) when they invite me to dinner.
~ Caterers outdo competition by making party food delicious, rather than nutritious, and vegetables are not at the top of their lists.
~ Vegetables rarely accompany ballpark hotdogs or pepperoni pizza.
~ Too often the best a restaurant has to offer in the vegetable department is two spears of asparagus and a small sprig of parsley.

Non-vegetable foods are highly palatable, aggressively advertised, and easily available.[27]

~ In our often "meat-centric" society, the steak or the pork chop is the centerpiece of the meal. Vegetables are an afterthought, and usually less-than-healthful fried potatoes or overcooked frozen peas.
~ Even the salad bar is normally a nutritional wasteland, offering little more than iceberg lettuce, fattening croutons, and cholesterol-laden dressing. (And don't forget those ubiquitous "bacon-flavored" artificial bacon bits . . . guess where that "bacon-flavor" comes from? No surprise here: chemicals!)

> **Sometimes the most effective and seemingly simplistic choices are the most difficult to carry out. Our main cues for food choice are habit and easy accessibility.**

Despite my nutrition acumen, I don't care how many grams of trans fat or oxidized fat a blueberry muffin contains at any hungry moment – especially if that muffin is within reach and the carrot sticks aren't. I might eat the muffin even if I'm not hungry!

Much of our food promotes pleasure rather than health![28]

Has it ever been different? In 1844, Ralph Waldo Emerson said: "Let the stoics say what they please, we do not eat for the good of living, but because the meat is savory and the appetite is keen."[29]

It's no wonder that adherence to our somewhat laughable *Dietary Guidelines for Americans* has had little if any benefit in preventing major chronic disease.[30] A surprising statement in a special article in the *New England Journal of Medicine,* titled "Cancer Undefeated," points out that "prevention is likely to be more difficult and costly than treatment."[31] A frightening philosophy indeed.

Perhaps some distant day the ballpark vendor will sell red and green peppers stuffed with pine nut spinach salad, steamed broccoli, or walnut-sprinkled wild sprouts, instead of (or at least along with) popcorn, hotdogs and pretzels. But right now, when it comes to vegetables, we appear to be stuck – cradled in custom, despite what we know. It is obvious that a new approach is needed.

The encouraging news is that there are a few innovative and remarkably user-friendly food-type supplements now available to help compensate for what the flight attendant plunks down in front of you. One such product in particular is in my purse or briefcase at all times.

MY OWN HEALTH JOURNEY

It has been more than fifty years since I started my quest for nutrition information, but it could have been yesterday – not only because of my vivid memories in search of what I needed to eat to bear healthy children, but also because decades later it appears that so little progress has been made. Once I found out what worked, I tried to share that knowledge with friends and family. In the 1940s, I might as well have been baying at the moon nightly.

I could not understand why so few would listen – why my husband and I were considered "off the wall" for merely suggesting that what you feed a child has to do with the health of that child.

But now I am wiser. I know that to change things is never popular, especially when it comes to dietary habits. More than that, my message implied that we were responsible for our own health, and if disease has already set in, the guilt is hard to accept.

Equally significant, I know how difficult it is to give up a present pleasure for a future benefit – even if you are falling apart!

> Human behavior is no doubt the biggest killer of all. (Think about this: The number one cancer killer is lung cancer. We know it is primarily caused by smoking, yet it remains at the top of the cancer list even today.)

In the early days, you had the social status of a wet mop if you took supplements or refused a sweet dessert. Carrying bottled drinking water was certain to limit party invitations. However, as the years have passed, I've witnessed a lot of my early critics change their thinking, now doing exactly what my family had been doing for years. But mind you, for major change I had to wait more than half a century . . . and we still have a long way to go.

I've seen how bad things were, and how much they've improved. And I can tell you with firm conviction that our greatest progress has been in *immune enhancement.* The full understanding and widespread knowledge of the strength of immunity as we know it today is very recent knowledge. Given the right substances (that is, specific nutrients), we can keep our immune system at peak efficiency, so that harmful, unsolicited squatters simply do not proliferate, nor do they become more serious troublemakers.

> For optimal health, we cannot lose our rapport with nature. Only that which is natural will keep our immune system working at its efficient best.

Today, there is increased awareness that real medical progress did not come from drugs or genetic engineering or double-blind, randomized, placebo-controlled, cross-over designs – too many of which, when carried across the threshold of research into the real world – have been far too protracted on promise and woefully wanting in results. There is a vast difference between "significant" statistics and the person who is actually sick.

We learned from our past that a predominant micronutrient such as beta-carotene, when taken out of context and packaged into a pill, is *not* a magic bullet that can be used to replace food. In fact, a combination of many different factors – including groups of compounds such as flavonoids or plant sterols – probably contribute in a small way to the overall benefits of fruit and vegetables.[32]

Even among the alternative practitioners there is much to be learned. Good health means more than swallowing isolated vitamins. Many single-substance supplements, although of value for certain therapeutic measures, provide a blunt tool for the highest level of wellness. By the turn of the millennium, we learned that for every nutrient discovered to be essential for optimum health, there are many more not yet isolated. More importantly, we now understand that one nutrient is dependent on another, almost ad infinitum.

Roger Williams, the distinguished biochemist who was so far ahead of his time with contributions to modern nutritional science, was the first to point out that: *The need for phenylalanine is decreased if tyrosine is supplied, the need for methionine is decreased if cystine is supplied, and the need for tryptophane hinges in part on how much niacinamide is in the diet.*

To this day, the analytical approach has not yet been able to tell us *everything* about how the molecular pieces are integrated. It's so much more than a matter of food breaking down into component parts, and there are still many secrets kept hidden from us.

The absurdity of medical advice was epitomized recently in an announcement that children suffer more cavities because they are drinking non-fluoridated bottled water. Never mind the initial causes of cavities. Never mind that children are getting plenty of fluoride from other sources (it abounds in tap water served in restaurants, canned foods, bottled juices, sodas, restaurant foods, soups, and so on). Never mind that fluoride is a useless waste product of industry, turned golden egg through propaganda and false conclusions of the business-minded geese.

Or how about this "brilliant" finding: "The increasing prevalence of childhood asthma could in part be accounted for by the decreased use of aspirin among pediatric patients."[33] Do you smell an aspirin company marketing team in that research lab at all?

Progress has various emissaries. As for nutrition history, the good news is that a series of products on hand today have a remarkable impact on your immune system, and are currently playing a major role in the early success of immunotherapy. Their discoveries, although now validated scientifically, did not necessarily have their beginnings with trained researchers or doctors. In fact, many of them have been around for thousands of years!

These products – with emphasis on one in particular and its effects on your immune system – are what this book is about.

This book is intended to do two things:

1) explore the basics of the science of immunity and nutrition within which the nutrients in young barley leaf work

2) serve as a practical guide for nutraceutical supplementation

Whatever health program our country adopts, none can make you healthy if you don't look after yourself. The lack of progress in circumventing critical illness should be no surprise: *Only one-third of one percent of health expenditure has been used for prevention in the United States in recent years.*[34] Ironically, advanced countries like ours, consuming the largest portion of resources on medicine, can be counted among those with the *highest* numbers of people living with the fear of serious disease.

Too many times I hear the refrain, "I eat well and I exercise, and yet I get sick." The tenets widely espoused as "prevention" suggest an involvement with low-fat foods, jogging, and learning to think good thoughts.

The fact that this advice has not changed the incidence or altered the outcome of the majority of our country's medical problems is finally sinking in.

But you are already halfway there, having opened the pages of this book. When you are finished, and when you begin to make the simple lifestyle changes you are soon to learn about, you will be safely on the road to your new health destiny. It may be the most important thing you ever do for yourself, and hopefully one day far in the future, when you are old and gray and rocking away happily in your rocking chair (rather than being cared for and fed by by an orderly at the care center), you will think back to the day you decided to take your life into your own hands . . . and I hope you will smile knowingly.

When my first book, *The Kamen Plan for Total Nutrition During Pregnancy*, was published in 1981, I received a letter from the American Medical Association. The letter warned that I should be more responsible about my messages. How dare I suggest - the letter stated - that one vitamin, folic acid, could actually prevent birth anomolies? Now, of course, they want to put that nutrient in our cereals, to be sure we all have an ample supply.

When the first edition of my book, *Hormone Replacement Therapy, Yes or No: How to Make an Informed Decision,* was published in 1992, I had to answer to a few very important upper level agencies about my claims that adding synthetic progestin increases the risk of breast cancer. Fortunately, I had the documentation to back up my statements. Isn't it sad the the research had gone unnoticed by those who could have spared so many women so much misery (and even death) - until recently?

CHAPTER TWO
BEYOND VITAMINS:
The Next Level of Supplementation

...in which we explain nutraceuticals and functional foods: what they are, what they do, and why the body needs them.

THE WAY WE WERE: DIETS OF DAYS PAST

The Neolithic lifestyle would have been the envy of the most rigorous personal trainer and nutritionist of today. At that time, human beings consumed nothing but vegetables fresh from the vine, fruit picked from the trees, and fresh-killed wild game. They chewed on bone marrow and antler and ate organ meats. They caught fish from unpolluted water. Their diet was organic and fresher than anything available in any supermarket today. Exercise was a natural part of everyone's day, and with no artifical light, aside from a flickering fire, they got lots of sleep. Very few were afflicted with heart disease, cancer, diabetes, or arthritis. Of course, those who lived more than 10,000 years ago were not necessarily in better health than we are today. There were droughts, famines, and food shortages that challenged the resourcefulness of these people, sometimes forcing them to undertake long migrations or face starvation. *But their problems did not originate with the food they ate.*

Can we duplicate the good health experienced by the Neolithics when times were good? We can't. However, we can get close. Let's start with our modern diet, work backwards, and see what kind of changes we would have to make to return to the natural food environment for which our bodies are so perfectly designed.

20 Years Ago

First, let's wind the clock counterclockwise just a decade or two, to the time before the advent of our new genetically modified foods. This eliminates the new synthetic proteins and the new, hard-to-diagnose allergies that may be associated with them.

> **Selecting non-genetically modified foods is not a difficult step to take, and it will become easier if current efforts to label such foods are successful.**

75 Years Ago

Next step: we go back to the first half of the twentieth century, prior to a time when food engineering, frozen foods, additives like hydrogenated vegetable oil, MSG, and corn syrup sweeteners became all too common. This is more difficult – it means we have to buy most of our groceries at the health food store. (And even there we need to do some careful label reading.)

But we can avoid most of the witch's brew of additives thrown into food products for color, taste, shelf life, and "mouth feel." With just a little effort, we can also do without the enzyme-depleted frozen preparations that are all too common in the modern diet, made available to us at about the same time (mid-twentieth century).

> **To encourage us to make such changes, let's keep in mind that science has yet to find any method of preservation comparable to that of nature.**

125 Years Ago

Now we flip the calendar back to the late nineteenth century. No chemical pesticides and no synthetic fertilizers here! More than a hundred years ago, the density of the barnyard and the poultry farm was much lower, so infections were less likely to spread among the animals. Consequently, there wasn't as much need for antibiotics for livestock or chickens, even if these drugs had been available. Artificial growth hormones had not yet been invented. There was also less monoculture, with crop rotation and natural pest management more the standard practice. So the need for pesticides was nowhere near what it is today.

It was also around this same time that we started adding chlorine to drinking water, which we now know causes calcium to be excreted.

We can duplicate a lot of this today: Shop for organic produce, meat, and poultry at the farmer's market, and learn about the methods used at the farms that produce your food. And of course, drink chlorine-free bottled or filtered water.

200 Years Ago

Now go back two hundred years, to the pre-industrial society of the early nineteenth century. No railroads; no refrigeration. Ice is expensive. Nearly every community has to produce most of its own food locally. The much shorter distribution path from farm to dinner plate means that food is fresher, and only available in season. At this point in time, food preservation in the American kitchen is a basic housekeeping skill.

The food quality was high, but look at how much work we had to do! Not all technology degrades food, and it is much easier to run a self-sufficient farm today. But few of us are ready to drop that far out of our industrial society and start milking cows or plowing fields.

So we must rely even more heavily on the farmer's market, the health food store, and our backyard vegetable garden to recapture some of the high quality and freshness of locally grown food.

Then: Local farm → basket → table

Now: Commercial farm → silo → truck → processing plant → truck → storage plant → railroad → distribution warehouse →truck → supermarket → car → refrigerator →table.

2,000 Years Ago

As we go back farther through the pre-industrial centuries, we find relatively little change. Earlier cultures tended to rely more on fish and fish products than we do now. This can be duplicated because some ocean fish are still wild, organic, and "free range." (Select carefully, though: Fish contamination is already so high that eating fish exposes 1 in 4 pregnant women to levels of mercury that could threaten the developing fetus.[1])

Ancient people also ate far more animal organ meats than we do. Not too many of us have a taste for brains, kidneys, or spleens. Even if we could find quality organic organ meats (most can no longer be sold legally), this is where many of us draw the line.

10,000 Years Ago

Are we there yet? Not at all.

Two thousand years ago people had already made cereal grains the "staff of life," much to our nutritional detriment. But in the very early days of agriculture, the grains were genetically natural, not yet modified by extensive selection and crossbreeding. So we will wind our clock back to a time *before* our hypothetical farmer of 10,002 years ago (described in our introduction) to an era that predates the discovery of genetic engineering and the beginning of the modern hexaploid grains.

Luckily we can still buy ancient grains, barley being one of the best. But avoiding foods made with modern commercial wheat is more difficult. With effort, however, it can be done.

20,000 Years Ago

Even the people of 10,000 years ago were not always feeding their bodies what was needed most.So now we will go back *another* 10,000 years or so, to the Paleolithic era.

No agriculture. No cereal grains. No dairy products. No stale food transported over long distances. No preservatives, pesticides, hormones, antibiotics or hydrogenated vegetable oils. All food was fresh and wild. We ate "cereal" as grasses, not as grains. This is a big improvement – cereal grasses have approximately fifty times the vitamin and mineral density of grains.

We don't really know to what extent cereal grasses were part of the ancient diet. We suspect that early humans used stone tools to break up the fiber or to extract therapeutic juices from grasses, just as many of us do today with powered juicing machines.

150,000 Years Ago

Have we finally gone back far enough to glimpse the ideal food environment? Not yet.

150,000 years ago people started using fire to cook food. Fire made it possible to make foods more palatable, to disguise off-taste, and to keep some foods for longer periods of time. But fire introduced cancer-causing oxidized fats and oils. Fire also destroys food enzymes and vitamins.

A strong case can be made that it was really the discovery of fire and cooking that started human health on its long downhill slide.

Some people make a sincere effort to duplicate the raw Paleolithic diet, but it requires a level of dedication few of us will ever have. Many interpretations of this diet involve a strict vegetarian or vegan regimen.

While there may be therapeutic benefits to a raw vegan diet, the anthropological evidence suggests that the human diet has always included some animal protein. No strictly vegan aboriginal culture has ever been found. So while the "raw food" diet is usually practiced as a "raw vegan" diet, a more accurate and authentic Paleolithic regimen would be raw, non-vegan, and would also consist of fish and wild game – including all parts of the animal, *especially* the organs.

500,000 Years Ago

Perhaps we can blame our downhill slide on a simpler invention – the container! Half a million years ago people could only travel with what they could carry in their hands. There was no easy way to bring water to the cave, and nothing in which to store food. Most foods had to be eaten when and where found. Thus the container had a profound effect on human health, making it possible for hunter-*eaters* to become hunter-*gatherers*.

(No, they were not eating dinosaur meat. Dinosaurs disappeared from earth 65 million years ago.)

AND NOW, THE 21st CENTURY
AND THE ROLE OF FUNCTIONAL FOODS

As we snap back to our modern time, we recognize that it is virtually impossible to return to the food environment that would be in our best health interest. We can, however, infer some practical hints from studying this phase of human prehistory. It explains, for example, why our digestive system seems to be poorly adapted to drinking water (or any other liquid) along with a meal: before there were containers, a drink of water usually meant a trip to the river.

The prehistoric food environment also helps us understand the value of foods like fresh sprouts – foods that are live and growing even as you put them into your mouth. We thrive with optimum health on such foods, but how can we secure such a diet easily on a daily basis, given our current lifestyles?

This is where nutraceuticals and functional foods come in.

The best strategy is to select special foods and food supplements that embody most of the properties that are missing from even the most perfect and healthful modern diet.

Consider food enzymes. Nearly all natural foods come "pre-packaged" with many of the enzymes necessary to help with their own digestion. This is not because the plant is being considerate of human digestive needs; it is because our digestive system is programmed to make use of what it finds in whole natural foods.

Raw food is the most ideal way to obtain enzymes, since these foods provide the very enzymes needed for their own digestion. Each enzyme breaks down the substance it was made to handle, like a key that will fit only one lock.

The problem is that enzymes are very easily destroyed by stress, heat, light, time, and oxygen. In addition, airborne pollutants and and stimulant drugs like caffeine, can reduce the effectiveness of enzymes.[2] Our challenge is to start with the most enzyme-rich foods we can find – which usually implies fast-growing plants – and process and handle them in a way that preserves as much of the enzyme potency as possible. Young powdered barley leaf is a perfect example.

NUTRA *WHA TICALS*...?

What exactly are nutraceuticals? And what is the difference between a nutraceutical and a functional food?

A functional food is simply a special food selected because it provides a concentration of nutrients having a health benefit beyond providing essential nutrients.

Sometimes a functional food is a food to which something may have been added to increase its nutritional quality. (But be careful, as the term is also commonly applied to foods associated with claims that may be a long way from any form of accepted validation.)

Nutraceuticals are essentially the same as functional foods, although they tend to be more concentrated – more supplement-like than food-like. Foods processed in such a way as to render them more "practical" also fall into the nutraceutical classification.

There is a large area of overlap in the usage of the terms functional food and nutraceutical, and either can be applied to a wide range of products.

Brewer's yeast was one of the first and most traditional nutraceutical supplements available at health food stores. Even though brewer's yeast is usually sold as tablets or as a powder, the product itself is composed of whole yeast organisms, bursting with enzymes and vitamins and trace nutrients. Yogurt, on the other hand, is more likely to be classed as a functional food because it is more food-like than supplement-like. But it too contains complete organisms with their own complete sets of enzymes, vitamins, and trace nutrients.

Sprouts, vegetable juices, and some types of sauerkraut are other examples of functional foods, whereas dehydrated sprouts, velvet deer antler, stabilized rice bran, and colostrum are more likely to be called nutraceuticals.

Some nutraceuticals approach the boundary between nutraceuticals and isolated supplements. "Food-grown vitamins" are produced with the use of biological processes that generate supplements very rich in specific ingredients, and while they also contain many of the cofactors and trace nutrients of whole organisms, they are one step removed from nature's balance of ingredients.

Sometimes the use of these products is justified; sometimes it's better to stay with more natural forms. A lot depends on availability, cost, and purpose. For that matter, there are times when the use of a pure synthetic single ingredient is warranted, such as massive doses of vitamin C used in therapies against a number of disease conditions, or a large amount of vitamin A for just a short period of time to nip an oncoming cold in its tracks.

But specific nutrients rarely perform their own individual miracles independently. In its natural context, every recognized nutrient is escorted by a profuse array of poorly understood cofactors. So even when we use an isolated nutrient therapeutically, it serves us better if we are also endowed with a range of nutrients from more natural sources.

Nor have we discovered the most efficient delivery vehicle for the absorption and bioavailability of a lone, single nutrient.[3] All these facts are clues to the amazing performance of nutrient-rich whole foods when contrasted with stand-alone vitamins or minerals, regardless of how dominant a role that single nutrient may play in our metabolic processes.

The beneficial effects of isolated vitamins have always been difficult to demonstrate in population studies. But the positive worth of consuming foods that are high in these vitamins is very clear and easier to validate.

A huge outpouring of published data affirms that people who eat more of the *foods* containing the nutrients responsible for optimum health are more disease-resistant.[4,5,6,7,8]

Why should this be? Again, it's the unidentified cofactors, plus the freshness, the lack of destructive processing, and the natural delivery system.

One example of the difference between nutrient intake in supplemental form compared with food was demonstrated by a medical team at the University of Michigan. These experts examined levels of antioxidant consumption. They then compared rates of LDL oxidation (the potential health-reducing or "bad" cholesterol factor) and found that women who obtained vitamin E from their diet displayed significant reductions in unwanted LDL oxidation. This was not the case for women who took vitamin E as a supplement.[9] (Oxidation and antioxidants are explained in more detail in chapter 4.)

In another study reported in the *American Journal of Clinical Nutrition*, it was found that vitamin E in food was protective against death from stroke, but there was no such defensive property from simply supplemental vitamin E or other antioxidant vitamins.[10]

Nutrition is still an extremely inexact science. What we don't know about food and health far outweighs what we have thus far discovered. Recognition that we simply lack full understanding about our living cells and the deep matters of the human body has given us the reality check needed to start sending healers in new directions.

> America's rediscovery of the healing power
> of *plants* marks a return to an ancient form
> of medicine practiced for thousands of
> years – and one that is still practiced today
> by 80 percent of the world's people.

That's why it makes sense to rely on the way nature delivers nutrients to the body, as is the case with nutraceuticals and functional foods. And, as you will learn in subsequent chapters, that's why young barley leaf powder promises to be the best of the best.

I'LL SAY IT ONE LAST TIME – EAT YOUR VEGETABLES!

Dr. Yank Coble of the American Medical Association once said: *"In God we trust. All others must have data."* To confirm that the principles cited here are grounded in solid scientific research, note the following examples of studies showing how food is superior to supplements:

Specific nutrients do not always reduce chronic disease
Clinical trials have not always been as successful as food and diet in demonstrating that a specific nutrient supplement can substantially reduce risk for chronic disease.
> *Annals of the Review of Public Health*[11]
> *Journal of the American Medical Association*[12]

Spinach is better than supplemental vitamin C
Ten ounces of fresh spinach produced a greater rise in women's blood antioxidant scores than that caused by 1,250 milligrams of vitamin C.

"The participants in this study must have been absorbing other compounds in this vegetable," concluded a report in *Agricultural Research*.[13] Spinach is a fantastic vegetable, but ten ounces of fresh spinach would be many times more than the amount Popeye ate in one gulp. (It would, in fact, fill at least four of his spinach cans.)

Antioxidants in food combat cataracts better than isolated components
Dietary antioxidants can lessen our ever-increasing cataract problem by preventing oxidation within the lens. But an extensive study reported in *Epidemiology* shows that neither vitamin C, E or A could decrease the risk, and only moderate results are achieved with the use of lutein and zeaxanthin in supplemental form.

Present findings add support for recommendations to consume *vegetables* high in carotenoids or lutein daily. Spinach, kale, and broccoli are the most important contributors of lutein. Zeaxanthin is found in spinach and cabbage; carotenes in carrots.[14,15]

An apple a day . . . beats isolated vitamin C
About one serving (100 grams) of fresh apple provides antioxidant activity equal to that of 1,500 milligrams of vitamin C. But because the amount of vitamin C in an apple is only about 5.7 milligrams, almost all the antioxidant activity must come from a mix of the apple's phytochemicals. The researchers reporting in *Nature* say: "The key here is the combination of antioxidants in the apples. Apples contain almost 100 known phytochemicals – there is a synergy effect."[16] (This is why the supplement industry has begun to offer us a wide range of antioxidants.)

Carotenoids from food fight colorectal cancer
The positive benefits of vegetables against colorectal cancer is pronounced, even in advanced colorectal lesions, but the carotenoid extraction (alpha- and beta-carotene) contributes only marginally to the effects.[17] Only two parts of the carotenoids were used, rather than the whole complex of carotenoids.

Vitamin E is effective when used with other antioxidants
Past research shows that vitamin E is protective for heart disease. But recent experiments could not offer the same results, so scientists reporting in *New England Journal of Medicine* suggested that previous success was due to high intakes of *other* antioxidants and micronutrients taken with the vitamin E supplement.[18]

To add to the complexity of the issue, *Nutrition Reviews* reminds us that vitamin E deficiency can cause suppression of the immune response system, and that the American diet is acutely deficient in vitamin E.[19] Vitamins and minerals can also have very different effects – sometimes negative, and sometimes positive, depending on the type of nutrient and the level of intake.[20]

Here are a few additional illustrations that may surprise you.

Vitamin A
Vitamin A compounds can sometimes enhance and sometimes inhibit the growth of malignancies.[21]

Iron
Excess iron can turn vitamin C into a *pro*-oxidant instead of an antioxidant, so instead of preventing free radical damage, it may contribute to it. Some studies indicate that excess iron can be a factor in joint pain, especially in the hip, and can cause a variety of symptoms from hair loss to heart flutters. The same type of fatigue characteristic of too little iron may be experienced with too much iron.

Genistein
Genistein is one of the active ingredients in soy, extracted from the whole product. Test animals consuming genistein had offspring with decreased birth weight and early onset of puberty in males.[22] Results are entirely different when the supplements are

made of whole soy. Apparently, genistein requires the wholeness of soy for its remarkable effectiveness, especially beneficial when this bean is organic (hard to come by, however), and in the sprout stage.

Calcium
If large amounts of calcium are ingested in supplemental form, your body turns off its production of the important vitamin D hormone, stopping the bone-remodeling process. The result is an unhealthy skeleton.[23] [[expand]]

High-dose Multivitamin Caveat
Very high-dose multivitamin supplements promoted the development of fibrosis (the formation of fibroids), and prevented beneficial remodeling of coronary plaque composition. (The doses used in this Canadian cardiovascular study included 30,000 IU of beta-carotene.)[24]

Clearly, vitamins alone will never be the solution to our modern health problems. Effective preventive medicine demands more complete tools. Great advancements in medicine have been made in the development of high-tech diagnostic methods.

Unfortunately, identifying afflictions has done very little to reduce their number! We are not yet all that good at preventing disease and preserving health.[25]

The complete safety and clear effectiveness of green plants explains why these products are fast becoming the most frequently self-prescribed dietary additions, rivaling the familiar vitamins and herbs. The health benefits of food-based supplements such as barley leaf promise to be far-reaching, and more evidence piles up each day that they are truly the key to health, longevity, and a super-charged immune system.

CHAPTER THREE
OUCH!
YOU CUT YOUR FINGER

...in which we discuss how your body knows what to respect and what to reject, as well as green leaf barley immune system-enhancing abilities.

Ouch! You cut your finger while slicing onions. Nothing serious, it's happened before. So you won't be surprised if the wound hurts for a little while, or gets a bit red or swollen.

You don't pay much attention to it beyond taking a simple precaution to prevent infection – perhaps some antibiotic ointment and a Band-Aid you found in the medicine cabinet. You vow to be more careful next time. You have no reason to be concerned with the details of the wondrous defense system your body is launching at this very moment towards the combat zone at the tip of your finger. Four-star generals can only dream of orchestrating such sophisticated tactical maneuvers.

We will describe a mere smattering of what takes place on the killing fields of your cut. Cursory as this explanation is, it will clarify just how it is that nutrients affect your health and well-being – especially those found in nutraceuticals like the young barley leaf.

The mechanics of this immune response apply to episodes as trivial as a simple surface injury or as life disrupting as a degenerative disease.

WHAT IS IMMUNITY ANYWAY?

Immunity is often thought of as the process by which you are protected against infection. This is certainly true, but your immune system has vastly more far-reaching effects on your overall health. Destroying invading meddlers is just a small part of what it can do.

> Your immune system can control inflammation and swelling. It can alter your body temperature. It can isolate and remove damaged or cancerous cells. And it can even protect you against toxins in the environment, a role that is more and more important in today's industrialized world.

Your immune system can also "remember." If you had chickenpox as a child, you probably won't get chickenpox again. You might get the mumps, but you are considered to be immune to the organism that causes chickenpox. This biological memory is contained as a chemical record in special white blood cells in your body – a marvelously complex process.

In its effort to select and attack "foe" and to avoid careless extermination of "friend," the immune system can also be nonspecific in what it goes after. That is, it need not be dependent on remembering a particular microorganism, as with chickenpox. It has controls to keep out unwanted foreign material in general, to recognize and destroy "other," even altered or damaged "self," without hurting healthy self, regardless of prior exposure.

As smart as your immune system may appear to be, it often makes grave mistakes. Allergies are examples of such mistakes, the result of an immune response overreacting to stimulation. This would not be a problem except for the fact that the stimulus is often far less harmful than the exaggerated response.

Another kind of immune system mistake is when "self" is mistaken for "other" and attacked. This is called an *autoimmune response* and there are at least forty known autoimmune diseases.[1] Arthritis is an example of an autoimmune disorder, the result of an immune response over-reacting to stimulation.

Autoimmune diseases are poorly diagnosed because the onset can be stealthy, and initial symptoms are often non-specific – tiredness, fatigue, or fever. In addition to arthritis, caused by immune-based inflammatory responses that destroy joint tissue, note these other diseases cited as immune-system errors:

Diabetes – thought to be the result of damage to the pituitary gland, initiated by an immune response in early childhood[2,3] (Autoimmune type 1 diabetes is the most common of all chronic diseases of children[4])

Cardiovascular disease – the heart becomes the target organ for an initial episode of myocardial damage, triggering an autoimmune response[5,6]

Cancer – clear failure of the immune system to effectively deal with the proliferation of damaged cells

Multiple sclerosis – tissues of the central nervous system are mistakenly attacked

Thyroid disease (includes Hashioto's thyroiditis and Graves' disease) – frequently developed problem following delivery, caused by an immune rebound mechanism after birth[7]

Anemia – antibodies are directed against bone marrow[8]

Myasthenia gravis – endocrine glands are affected

Lupus – connective tissues are assaulted

Endometriosis – mucous membranes of the uterus are effected[9]

As we look deeper into the role of the immune system, we see that a large portion of many other degenerative diseases may also be caused by immune-system downfalls or deficiencies. If we can understand how to improve our immune system, we can understand how to greatly improve our health and longevity.

THE BATTLE BENEATH THE SKIN

Let's look at the immune strategies activated when you cut your finger with that wayward kitchen knife. Just as expected, the wound area became red and inflamed, and the site of the injury became swollen and sore to the touch.

Many of the cells in or on your body are not your own. Your skin is home to about twenty million bacteria on every square inch. But your skin is your first defense against pathogens. Chemicals in your perspiration and the oils you secrete inhibit some of the harmful bacteria, while encouraging the growth of other "friendly" bacteria that provide stiff competition for unwanted guests.

The acidic nature of your skin secretions prevents large classes of pathogens from entering.

In addition, there are chemicals present on your skin that dissolve the cell walls of many kinds of microbes.

You are pretty well protected...*that is, until you cut yourself!* Once that happened, some of these parasites took advantage of the new inroads created by your cut and quickly slithered in to greener pastures – deeper layers, where treasured nutrients are far more bountiful than on your skin's surface. But...not to worry!

A patrolling immune cell, called a macrophage, prowls through your inner tissues, 24-7. Its job is to engulf any intruder it happens upon. But that's a textbook response. Such policing may actually happen on occasion, but all too often the intrusive bacteria multiply manyfold, far outnumbering the watchdog macrophages. Not unlike successful territorial invasions, the trespassers victimize the defenseless residents of your body – your cells and tissues.

With their increased progeny, the enemy thinks nothing of injuring anything that gets in its way. You need more than a passing vigilante macrophage or two for protection. So your abused cells emit SOS signals in the form of chemical secretions.

> **Blood vessels answer a call for help by expanding their walls and becoming more porous. More fluid can now accumulate, which is why your wound feels warm and turns red.**

As additional blood flows to the area, the molested tissue swells and becomes more sensitive. It's all part of the inflammatory response: The swelling puts pressure on nerve endings, a sign for the rest of your body to respect the disturbed area and protect it from further damage. An elevation in body temperature is also triggered. That's why swelling, inflammation, and fever are typical responses to infection.

Within an hour, the first regiment of soldiers is dispatched – this time it's the neutrophils. The increased size of the holes in the capillary walls makes it easier for neutrophils to reach the scene of the infection. A great battle is underway. The foes, however, are well armed, their toxic weapons deadly. But again, no cause for concern! Your protectors, the neutrophils, are able to imprison the enemy. It's a suicide mission, however – in the process, these warriors will die protecting you.

Since the lifespan of the neutrophil is brief (it can only devour just so many bacteria before its demise), reinforcements soon arrive – not only more neutrophils by the tankload, but also longer-lasting allies, the macrophages. Like microscopic bulldozers, these macrophages must use some of their own enzymes to cut through the jungle of fibers, protein, and debris that has accumulated at the war zone.

Finally at the scene, the macrophages wrap finger-like projections around the bacteria and devour them, sealing the intruders' doom with more of their digestive enzymes.

> Luckily, the macrophage has a proverbial hollow leg – an insatiable appetite. After devouring one enemy, it hastily starts another meal, eliminating one adversary after another.

Now for the *really* interesting part. The after-dinner antics provided by the macrophages are ingenious: These defending cells display the identifying "thumbprint" of the invader on their own surface – actually, a chemical message for assistance, in the form of helper T cells. The T cells, in turn, respond by multiplying. By releasing additional immune cells, the protective military force is increased.

Some of the T cells radio to other cells, called B cells, which connect up with the bacteria, and now *they* begin to reproduce. A number of B cells record the information, which help your body fight the same kind of bacterium should you encounter it again at a later date. (Memory cells can remain circulating in your blood and lymphatic system for many years. Next time the same pathogen shows its face inside your body, your immune system will be able to respond more quickly and more efficiently.) Other B cells join the fight, emitting thousands of antibodies each second.

Most antibodies work in a surprisingly simple way. They have surface proteins that exactly fit the surface proteins of the bacteria. This causes the bacteria to lock together, as if handcuffed by the antibody. Now additional immune cells don their chef hats and whip the bacteria into a tasty dessert for the macrophages. Or they may annihilate the bacteria by viciously puncturing their cell walls. Either way, it's death for the attackers.

> **War victims (dead tissues, digested microorganisms, spent immune cells, and cellular debris) may seep from the wounded area in the form of *pus*.**

Now that the enemy is vanquished, the wounded area is finally ready for repair and for healing.

The example cited here refers to just a minor cut, an abridged version at that. Imagine how your body works to keep you free of more serious invasions! Superficially, many pathogens look just like human cells. Which ones should be destroyed, and which ones need to be protected?

There is an incomprehensibly large number of different forms of living material in your blood and tissue, and these self/other decisions must be made continuously and automatically. If we had to make these minute-by-minute assessments for our own immune system, we wouldn't give ourselves very good odds for even short-term survival. I would have better luck landing a space shuttle than running my own immune system.

If we had to understand the instructions for manufacturing antibodies to fight pathogens, even if we could identify them, we'd be in even more trouble. These molecules are huge – comprised of thousand of atoms and amino acid combinations – and if just one amino acid is wrong, the molecule won't fit the target and the antibody is worthless.

We've already cited examples of immune systems that *over-re-act*. An *under-reacting* immune system can be just as devastating – the other end of the spectrum.

A cancer cell may get your immune system to ignore its ominous presence by hiding behind some protein, or disposing of its antigenic calling card, or even mutating so that it looks like something else. All it takes is one cell aberration escaping detection.

How much do we really know about what the immune system sees? How it sees? How it distinguishes nonself from healthy self? What a tumor does when under attack? The use of the immune system to treat disease has made steady (but not spectacular) headway over the past century.

Although the medical community refers to epidemics, even on a global scale, disease is really very personal – you and your body alone against illness.

Fortunately we all have this intricate defense system that turns out these astounding antibodies without our even being conscious of the events in progress. It is sophisticated, coordinated, and syncopated...and it's a good thing it's running on autopilot!

But what about when the system fails?

And what are the catalysts that initiate beneficial results?

Success in warding off long-lasting infection is dependent on several important factors, among them the efficiency of your immune system to deal with nonspecific responses.

And that immune competence is totally dependent on the presence of very specific nutrients!

GREEN LEAF BARLEY AND IMMUNITY

The nutrients found in the young green barley leaf (and a small handful of other quality nutraceuticals) are immune-system enhancers. They help to facilitate the action-packed drama we just described. To understand the consequences of nutrient deficiencies, it's important to have at least a brief understanding of how these various details fit together.

Nutritional status and immune status are closely linked.[10] It is important to remember that your immune system does not do well with just one branch of the armed forces: it won't function with optimum efficiency with just the army, only the navy, or simply the marines or air force acting alone. Don't ever accept the hype that one single nutrient can be enough. Optimum health requires the combined efforts of the full gamut of protectors, all working together. Endless research confirms that these nutrients must come from whole food complexes. *Nature knows better than we do!*

We must not be misled by the fact that scientists can produce isolated nutrient deficiencies in laboratory animals. In contrast, human malnutrition is almost always a syndrome of multiple nutrient deficiencies. That's one reason we recommend nutraceuticals like the young green barley leaf, which is much better able to meet the nutritional requirements of your immune system than any single isolated (and often synthetic) nutrient.

Furthermore, many nutrients and their impact on immune status have yet to be explored. You certainly have a better chance of getting these nutrients in a nutrient-dense food-type supplement than in any bottle containing only a specific list of isolated nutrients.

Even marginal deficiencies of some nutrients are associated with impaired immune function. On the other side of the coin, function can also be disturbed when the concentration of a trace element is too *high*. High levels of vitamin E, for example, may suppress immune responses. Natural substances provide security against this kind of overdosing.

Here are just a few examples of how some of the nutrients in the young green barley leaf relate to immune competence:

~ *Vitamin E* is critical for proper function of the immune system.[11] Almost every action of the immune system has been shown to be altered by vitamin E intake – from resistance to infection, to antibody responses.[12] Moderate amounts of vitamin E can increase antibody production, with several studies showing increased immunocompetence.[13] Vitamin E is found in the membranes of immune cells as protection against oxidative damage.[14,15]

~ *Carotenoids* can be precursors to vitamin A, which is absolutely essential for immune function.[16]

~ *Iron* is essential to immunity. Iron deficiency can significantly impair immune responses.[17] Iron deficiency generally impairs host defenses and increases infection morbidity.[18]

~ *Beta-carotene* has been shown to have a variety of immune-enhancing effects, including increased resistance to immunogenic tumors. Beta-carotene stimulates natural killer immune cell activity.[19]

Nutraceuticals function as a first-aid kit for your immune system, helping to bolster its effectiveness and to choreograph its specialized cells in your best health interest.

Think of these nutrients as a healthy dose of Congressional defense spending – a worthwhile investment to keep your body's forces fully armed and at the ready. Your health – and your life – may one day depend on it.

INFECTIONS: EVER-PRESENT

We have only recently proven that microorganisms have a caus-
ative role in almost all chronic illness. Studies show that:

~ most peptic ulcers are caused by *Helicobacter pylori* infection
(Note: aspirin-induced gastric injury is more likely when H. pylori is present.[20])

~ bacteria are linked to increased risk of cardiovascular disease[21]

~ multiple sclerosis has been virus-induced in test animals[22]

~ the spread of infectious disease may be global warming's greatest medical threat[23]

~ pathogens accelerate atherosclerosis[24]

~ cross-sectional studies performed worldwide have shown that
hepatitis C virus (HCV) infection is linked with type 2 diabetes[25]

~ infertile men are more likely to harbor a particular virus in
their semen than men without an infertility history[26]

~ streptococcal infection has been linked to psychiatric disorders
in children[27]

~ prenatal malaria exposure has been linked to later asthma[28]

~ infection is strongly implicated in autoimmune disease[29]

~ evidence supports infection as a cause of childhood leukemia[30]

~ infection may be responsible for many refractory cases of inflammatory bowel disease[31]

Antimicrobial resistance continues to increase at an alarming rate.[32]

In addition to associating pathogens with familiar diseases, new infectious agents have come onto the scene. No surprise, given today's trends of greater reliance on imported foods, extensive international air travel, improper use of antibiotics (responsible for antimicrobial resistance), plus the resurgence of old foes like tuberculosis – all making prevention more important than ever before.

IMMUNE-SYSTEM VOCABULARY: A FEW IMPORTANT WORDS

Pathogen. Any substance or microorganism foreign to the body that causes disease. Some are microscopic; others visible to the naked eye.

Phagocytes. White blood cells that literally engulf and devour unwanted cells or pathogens. In fact, phagocytes are referred to as "eating cells." They have no trouble knowing which cells to kill. Phagocytes include neutrophils, macrophages, monocytes, and eosinophils.

Neutrophils. Phagocytes comprising the largest number of all white blood cells (abundant in your blood, but absent from normal tissue).

T-lymphocytes. White blood cells that are not effective until they receive final conditioning in the thymus gland. This is a recently discovered part of the immune system, located in the upper chest.

CHAPTER FOUR
MY MOTHER,
THE LATE-BLOOMING
NUTRITION GURU

...in which we discuss how Mom learned enough nutrition to turn her life around, and armed with a little knowledge, helped her friends to overcome a host of health problems.

My mother came to me when she was in her late sixties, complaining, "I'm tired of being tired; I'm sick of being sick. I'll do anything you say."

And she meant it. We sat down together, and I outlined a simple plan for her. She complied totally with my suggestions, and in just a matter of weeks Mom looked younger and felt better than she ever had in her life. Truly – I mean it – better than she ever had in her life! She'd been an anemic child, had difficult pregnancies, was always tired, and was even rushed to the hospital with a heart attack when in her forties. Nowadays she had a hiatal hernia, high blood pressure, impaired hearing, a dropped uterus, frequent respiratory problems, severe neuralgia pains in her arm and on the side of her head, and constant backaches.

This turn-about in her life did have one embarrassing side effect, however. At the supermarket, she'd pick up a bag of potato chips from another shopper's wagon, scolding: "You shouldn't eat anything that doesn't *grow* crispy. Don't you know those are really potato-flavored fat chips?"

Or, she'd pick up a tub of ice cream from someone's cart and warn: "I hope you won't eat this before bed. If you do, your blood sugar will go up and interfere with your growth hormone production, and that affects how you age. You don't want to look old before your time, do you, dear?" And she would even give some very sophisticated nutrition advice: "If you MUST have this sweet junk in the evening, promise me you'll have some fiber with it."

Worse, she once pointed to a rather huge pile of hot dogs and bologna packets sharing space in a shopping cart with a young child. Loud enough for the entire store to hear, she shouted:

"A child eating all those nitrites increases the risk of developing leukemia! You should be reported for child abuse."

She addressed a poor bachelor in a gentler tone, his cart filled with ready-to-microwave hamburger patties: "I hope you know, sir, that 99 percent of our animals get hormone pellets placed in their ears. That makes them grow fatter *faster*, to say nothing of the herbicides, fungicides and pesticides lacing the grains the animals eat! Residues of those hormones and poisons find their way into that very meat you're buying today."

Is it any wonder her bridge partners kept saying, "No, Claire, we don't need a fourth this week. Maybe next time."

It seemed as if there was only one thing Mom hadn't learned: People have to be ready to accept this kind of information and, more importantly, *ready to make changes*. In our world of information overload, most people are generally aware of what's good for them and what isn't. We've all heard more than we care to know about fiber and calcium and how Grandma knew what she was talking about when she told us to eat our vegetables. Even *antioxidant* is becoming a household word. But we are also stuck in lifestyles and environments that are not the least bit conducive to eating five (in fact, now they're telling us we need *seven* and maybe even *nine*) portions of vegetables every single day for optimum health.

That's why I started Mom on special nutraceuticals before attempting to change her diet and before getting her involved in an exercise program. I used Aristotle's philosophy of *giving* before *taking away*. Translating that to table talk, it's much easier, for example, to get someone to add a packet of young barley leaf powder to their glass of water or juice than it is to get someone to completely overhaul their diet overnight. And even though more and more meals are eaten out these days, it's easy to take a nutraceutical packet along with you to the restaurant.

Aristotle's philosophy worked! Mom soon began to accept the fact that her body – even at her advanced age – had amazing curative powers when given the "right stuff." Now that she was ready to learn more, I loaded her up with books and articles.

OXIDATION: AN EXPLANATION

Mom's first probing questions raised my eyebrows. She asked, "Isn't oxidation a vital process? Isn't oxidation the means of supplying power to all our organs and muscles? Isn't oxidation the primary way we turn food into energy?"

"Yes, yes, and yes," I answered, after recovering from the shock of her inquisitive interest and newfound knowledge. "Then why is oxidation harmful?" Mom asked.

Wow! Mom *was* reading the books I'd given her! I explained that despite the fact that oxidation is one of the most fundamental and necessary biochemical reactions in the body, not all oxidation is desirable. Life on earth began in an oxygen-free environment, and the design of our cells still reflects this heritage.

The structures within our cells that take advantage of oxygen's reactive power to produce energy are carefully isolated from the other parts of the cell that might be severely damaged by oxygen. Oxidation of the wrong substances at the wrong time can have a devastating effect on our health.

There are many real-life examples of oxidation that you can hold in your hand. Think of plastic that has become brittle and powdery with age or from exposure to sunlight – the molecules having been broken up by the oxidation process. Or an old rubber band that has lost its elasticity and strength, the rubber molecules now stuck together. Or those white socks, washed with too much bleach, a powerful oxidizing agent. The long fibers of cotton in the socks are broken apart by oxidation, and the socks tear to pieces when we try to slip them onto our feet. (We won't do that again.)

These are examples of transformations in chemical structure due to oxidation that we can see and feel. The changes that occur with our own chemistry would be just as apparent if we could hold our cell membranes in our hands.

Oxidants play a major role in a variety of disorders, and the sources of oxidants vary. They can be released by inflamed cells, or sucked in from the environment (as in pollution or tobacco smoke). In addition to acute, usually reversible reactions, numerous diseases are associated with long-lasting oxidant stress, including heart disease and respiratory problems like asthma.

Oxidation, in the strictly defined sense as used by chemists, is simply a reaction that results in removal of electrons from a molecule. Electrons are tiny electrically charged particles that surround each atom in a kind of "orbit."

"You mean like those pictures of atoms with the circles floating around them?" asked Mom.

Yes. Oxygen, because of its ability to attract additional electrons, is thought of as the most common and strongest oxidizing agent. But other substances, like free radicals produced by the oxidation of many biological substances, can do the same work. I could sense Mom's next question. "I know," she smiled, "that free radicals are not students who escaped from Berkeley. But what are they exactly?"

I answered slowly and carefully: When a long and elaborate molecule is broken apart by oxidation, it usually releases a new molecule called a free radical. *Free* because it is not bonded to another molecule, and *radical* to indicate, in the obscure language of chemistry, that it is electrically charged. In turn, this charged particle can oxidize other molecules in a kind of chain reaction. So only one oxidation event can destroy a huge number of molecules.

The trouble is, a free radical interrupts a substance from doing its designated job – like identifying or blocking a virus; maybe controlling the regeneration of skin tissue; perhaps repairing the damage that occurs in an artery wall; or participating in healing the cut you got from slicing those onions.

So you see that oxidation throws a large monkey wrench into a very complicated machine. Only one single oxidation event can start this chain reaction, affecting countless vital processes. It's like tapping the first domino in a long row of dominoes, or a single match burning down the entire forest.

Aside from breaking apart complicated organic molecules and membranes and rendering enzymes inoperable, oxidation can also damage fatty acids. The problem here is that altered fat changes its shape in unnatural ways. Food processing companies use this property to advantage, by engineering melting point and "mouth feel." (Hence the ubiquitous partially hydrogenated vegetable oil added to far too many less-than-healthful foods.)

These substance may fool your biochemistry into using them in initial phases of all kinds of biological process – from immunity to synthesis of sex hormones. But you can't fool all of your body all of the time. The eventual result is a serious compromise of your most delicate health-sustaining immune pathways.

Long protein molecules that make up your skin, tendons, and arteries sometimes bond to each other in undesirable ways after oxidation damage. The immediate result is usually a significant loss of flexibility and elasticity.

> Wrinkled skin is an example of long-term results of oxidation that you can see; a stiff joint demonstrates one that you can feel.

The free-radical theory, currently the most accepted theory for the cause of aging, offers an explanation of the basis of degenerative disease because of the ability of free radicals to injure cells. Free radical damage has been scientifically validated in many diseases, including atherosclerosis, ischemia, Parkinson's disease, cataracts, many cancers, and rheumatoid arthritis.[1]

> The good news is that informed, nutrition-oriented practitioners have made use of two powerful tools:
> 1.) the reduction of oxidative stress in a patient's food and environment
> 2.) the increase of a supply of supplemental antioxidants to cope with the stress

Knowledgeable health-care advisors understand that nature has developed a complex set of interactive antioxidant systems as protection against oxidation. It is obvious that the second course of action (supplementation) is easier to come by and implement than the first, although the ultimate goal is to accomplish both.

MOM ASKS: WHAT IS AN ANTIOXIDANT?

And so, of course, the next question from Mom was: "What are antioxidants and how do they work?"

Ah! Now we get to the nitty-gritty.

> Antioxidants intercept toxins and other cancer-causing substances by rushing in and neutralizing the free radicals before they can do their damage to cell membranes and other tissues.

It's like me grabbing your hand before you tap that first domino. A molecule of one particular antioxidant, beta-carotene for example, can deactivate a single oxygen radical. A molecule of another antioxidant, vitamin C, can fight off two free radicals. Some enzyme systems, like superoxide dismutase, can deal with thousands of free radicals.

It turns out that a single antioxidant is seldom sufficient. These good guys work in teams, and no matter how much supplemental antioxidant you take of one kind, you still need an adequate supply of other antioxidants for optimal effect.

So antioxidants, if powerful and varied enough, intercept oxidation chain reactions. It has now been accepted that most diseases involve free radical reactions in tissue injury. Free radical reactions may be involved in multiple sites and at different stages of a chronic disease. But both acute and degenerative diseases involve free radical reactions in tissue injury. That's why there is so much emphasis on the importance of antioxidant intervention.

The concepts associated with antioxidants are critical to our understanding of health and disease because they provide the tools to really comprehend the difference between good meals and bad, to distinguish a healthful food preparation technique from a destructive one, and to identify an important and powerful supplement from one that may not be as effective or fast-acting.

"So something like the young green barley leaf that I have been taking has antioxidants?"

Absolutely. In fact, the green leaves of most plants have more antioxidants than other parts of the plant. The cells of green leaves require powerful protection from the onslaught of the sun.

Recall that health depends on more than one antioxidant system.

Mom was really paying attention. "What about the antioxidants that are added to food? I noticed when I followed your instructions to discard the boxes of cereal in my kitchen cabinet, BHT was listed in the ingredients to prevent oxidation. I know these cereals are 'dead' food, and that's why they don't attract bugs. But wouldn't the antioxidant – the BHT – be an advantage?"

The consensus among researchers is that artificial preservatives like BHT do far more harm than good. BHT is actually a *xenobiotic*, a harmful substance causing damage to bronchial and lung tissue. (The prefix *xeno* means foreign.)

Some time later, Mom came back with yet another question.

"My neighbor," she said, "wanted to know why I still take supplements since I am now so careful about what I eat. I told her that unless I could move to an unpolluted area up in the mountains, eat all my fruits and vegetables right from the vine or tree, and catch all my own fish and meat (and cook very little of it), I need to supplement with antioxidants. Is there anything else I should have said?"

Your answer was just fine, Mom.

There are many forms that antioxidant supplementation can take. Some foods and herbs, especially those considered to have *adaptogenic* properties, are high in natural antioxidants. By adaptogenic we mean a substance that has the ability to activate natural healing or immune responses. These substances stop their action when they are no longer needed, and thus bypass the negative side effects of artificial drugs. (In contrast, drugs continue their appointed job forevermore, causing unwanted side effects.)

Nutrients from adaptogenic foods or supplements also seem to somehow find the action sites where they are needed, without interfering with other physiological systems.

Functional foods are adaptogenic, and nutraceuticals are often prepared from functional foods.

A NEIGHBORHOOD OF HEALTH PROBLEMS ...SOLVED!

My mother lived in Forest Hills, a suburb of New York City, named for good reason. The street that Mom had to climb to get from her apartment to the shopping center was almost vertical! Great fun for the grandchildren when it snowed, but a journey that required frequent stops by most of the older folks, never mind those unfit members of the younger generation.

Mom called one day, more excited than I had heard her in a long time. "I climbed the hill today and didn't have to stop once!"

Remember our discussion about antioxidants, Mom? Among those found in green leafy vegetables are carotene, catechins, polyphenols, and vitamin E. Slowly, these antioxidants have been helping you to repair and replace previously damaged cells and tissues. You are becoming healthier, and you *should* be able to walk up that hill without stopping!

"All my neighbors have trouble walking up that hill. I'm going to start educating them."

I had visions of Mom standing on a street corner at the top of the hill, hawking her newfound nutrition knowledge and generously doling out leafy green nutraceuticals to every passerby. I should have known better. Instead, she asked me to prepare a summary of antioxidant benefits, validated in the medical literature. If I had papers on leafy greens in particular, so much the better. She would offer a few printed pages only to those who were interested. (Ah, she was learning!)

It turned out that almost all her friends expressed interest. They had been noticing how much better Mom was looking and feeling – the best selling point possible.

And then the anecdotes began rolling in...

Asthma
"Sarah said her diet change and supplements are helping her asthma. Is that possible?" Mom asked.

There's no question that reactive oxygen may be a contributing factor in patients with asthma.[2] Antioxidant nutrients are not absorbed efficiently in asthmatic patients even during the asymptomatic, or remission, periods of the disease.[3,4] It is accepted that the reduction in antioxidant intake over the last twenty-five years has been a factor in the increased prevalence of asthma.[5]

Patients with asthma generate increased amounts of reactive oxygen.[6] So you can see how antioxidants would be helpful. A Russian study provided evidence in favor of including antioxidants in combined therapy for bronchial asthma.[7]

In 1990, it was shown that the role of oxygen in airway disease had been largely neglected, and since antioxidant defenses are defective in asthma, it was predicted that "free radical scavengers" (as antioxidants are sometimes called) could play a useful role in therapy.[8]

I recalled that Sarah's grandchild also suffered from asthma and I told Mom to tell her that asthmatic children are also deficient in antioxidant protection, so supplementation is a good idea.[9] Several studies show that children suffering from bronchial asthma have disturbances in the oxidative-antioxidant balance.[10] Her granddaughter should certainly be taking nutraceuticals; the whole-food type are perfectly safe for children. Mixed with juice, these powders would be especially palatable for a young child.

Heart Health

Mom was full of other success stories. She related the improvement in Anne's LDL cholesterol – you know, the "bad" variety. Anne's LDL had been too high. LDL oxidation enhances its heart disease-causing factor, raising the possibility that antioxidants, which inhibit the oxidation of LDL, reduce the risk of coronary heart disease.[11]

Yet other studies also indicate that antioxidants can significantly decrease the risk for coronary heart disease.[12,13]

Emil Ginter, a renowned researcher whose groundbreaking work I have been following for many years, discussed a new concept of heart disease as it relates to the role of oxygen radicals. He concluded that the intake of antioxidants would, along with other corrective provisions, suppress the incidences of cardiovascular disease. High antioxidant vitamin levels in the blood are increasingly being associated with reduced risk of heart disease.[14,15]

Antioxidants can also inhibit platelet aggregation (the "sticking together" of blood platelets), and reduce atherosclerotic plaque.

"I know why you're emphasizing heart disease," Mom asserted. "It's the number one killer of both men *and* women." Yes, heart disease is responsible for one out of every three deaths, regardless of gender.

France and Finland have consistently had different coronary heart disease mortality rates, although the French and the Finnish have similar intakes of cholesterol and saturated fat. But the French also consume more plant foods – more vegetables (and thus, more antioxidants) – and so there are lower rates of heart disease mortality, in spite of the high intake of cholesterol and saturated fat![16,17]

Arthritis
Mom told me about Bernie's rheumatoid arthritis improvement. I told her that free radicals are implicated as causes of tissue damage in patients with this disease. It is possible, say the researchers, that antioxidants and free radical scavengers can provide protection. Results of studies are in line with the theory that a low antioxidant level is a risk factor for this disease.[18,19] And what prevents, may heal.

Clinical observations have already suggested that antioxidants may be beneficial for arthritic patients.[20]

It all makes sense, doesn't it? Rheumatoid arthritis and osteoarthritis are diseases in which there is progressive destruction of the joints. Active oxygen derived from various sources plays a role in this process, which may be influenced by appropriate treatment with antioxidants.[21]

Eczema
Mom told me about Bertha, whose eczema cleared up after green barley leaf supplementation. Not surprising! A Russian journal on dermatology reported that lipid peroxidation causes eczema.

> Get rid of the oxidation, and you get rid of the eczema.[22]

Lung disease

Bertha, encouraged by her success with the eczema clearing, asked Mom to ask about her daughter, who was a smoker. Oxidation of lung tissue can be prevented with antioxidants, thereby helping to prevent lung disease. (Although, of course, Bertha's daughter could best help herself by quitting smoking altogether.) The amount of antioxidants that offer protection always proves to be in excess of the current recommended dietary allowance.[23]

And cigarette smoking isn't the only factor in lung disease. Air pollution is predicted to be a major public health problem in all urban areas of the world.

Dementia

"I know that humor is an exaggeration of reality," Mom said philosophically one day. "We all tell these aging jokes about memory loss, but it's no exaggeration that 'losing it' is a major concern. I just read that our current rate of 360,000 cases of Alzheimer's disease each year will triple in the next few decades."

I explained that the role of oxidative stress in Alzheimer's disease is supported by a variety of studies. Mom jumped right in: "Antioxidants, then?" Yes!

> Higher dietary intakes of antioxidants were found to be associated with a lower risk of Alzheimer's disease.

Those with the highest intakes were 70 percent less likely to be afflicted. The results were based on a six-year study of more than five thousand men and women, aged 55 years and older. Similar results, however, were not observed with isolated synthetic forms of these nutrients.[24]

Cancer

And then came Mom's sad concern for her best friend: "What about Ruth?" Mom asked. "She has cancer, you know."

Mom, be careful about offering medical advice to people with serious conditions. If Ruth is receptive, you can help her learn as much as she can, and then she should discuss alternatives with her physician. Or you can help her find a physician who understands the value of nutritional modalities.

Ruth's doctor may already know that evidence implicates the involvement of oxygen-derived radicals in cancer development.

Mom helped Ruth prepare the following for her doctor:

~ Accumulation of DNA damage may contribute to cancer. Oxygen-derived radicals cause damage to membranes, mitochondria, proteins, lipids, and DNA.[25] Doctors may check on the level of lipid peroxides as a marker to discover cancer at an early stage. Amounts are correlated with advanced stages of cancer.[26] Since antioxidants help prevent these radicals from forming in the first place, many physicians use antioxidants as therapy, too.

~ Quercitin – part of a group of different compounds found in plant pigments – can help to fight cancer at its earliest stages by preventing changes in the cell that initiate cancer.[27]

~ The antioxidant vitamins decrease the incidence of pancreatic cancer.

All vitamins increase the activity of superoxide dismutase (SOD – explained in the next chapter) in pancreatic carcinomas.[28]

~ Treatment of small cell lung cancer cells with the antioxidant beta-carotene reduced cell proliferation.[29]

～ Dietary antioxidants protect against lung cancer.[30]

～ Pancreatic cancer cells stop growing with flavonoids.[31]

～ Over a hundred studies show a relationship of antioxidant intake or blood nutrient levels with cancer risk.[32]

～ Antioxidants are touted for the prevention of the recurrence of colorectal cancer. They lower recurrence of lesions and can be proposed as preventive agents.[33]

～ A twelve-year mortality follow-up of 3,000 participants showed that low antioxidant vitamin concentrations are associated with increased death from cancer of various sites (in the body).[34]

"These reports should impress her current physician," said Mom.

Diabetes
"Sarah's husband is diabetic; he looks and feels better since he's on leafy greens. That should impress her doctor, too."

Mom, you can tell Sarah's husband that diabetic patients tend to develop arteriosclerosis at an early age, and that oxidation of fats and proteins initiate its development. Antioxidants can therefore be helpful in staving off this condition. Sarah's husband should show his diabetologist the following three studies:

1. Oxidative stress resulting both from over-production of free radicals and the decreased efficiency of antioxidants, is now considered a factor in diabetic complications. Development of complications has also been atributed to oxidative stress. So the latest therapy aims at an increase in antioxidant defenses.[35]

2. Barley leaf extract may help to scavenge oxygen free radicals and inhibit LDL oxidation. This supplement may protect against vascular diseases in type 2 diabetic patients.

3. Oxidative damage is the major mechanism of diabetic cataracts.

Cataracts
"What causes cataracts anyway?" Mom asked, concerned about a common ailment in older people.

Cataract and macular degeneration are the two most important causes of visual impairment in seniors. Studies show that antioxidants protect against the effects that cause these conditions.

I showed Mom an excellent study that explained that the function of the eye lens is to collect and focus light on the retina. To do so, it must remain clear. Upon aging, lens constituents are damaged and precipitate in opacities, and we call these cataracts. The damage is due in part to light, and active forms of oxygen. Antioxidant nutrients appear to offer protection against cataracts

Researchers confirm that the ingestion of higher doses of antioxidant nutrients help to prevent the development of cataracts. Fifty million persons worldwide are blind due to cataracts, and in the United States alone there are 1.2 million cataract surgeries performed at an annual cost of over 3.2 billion dollars.

"Many of my friends are getting laser eye surgery. Too bad they didn't know about antioxidants way back when."

But they should know the value of antioxidants now. Ophthalmologists recommend antioxidant therapy for two weeks following laser surgery as it protects the cornea from the free radicals. At least 25 percent experience this problem, and they can benefit from the antioxidant supplementation.

"What about those who are just beginning to get cataracts?" Good question, Mom. The cataract effect of oxygen free radicals can be stopped by antioxidants, which are now considered useful for both prevention or therapy.

Aging
"I know I'm no spring chicken," Mom joked one day. "But don't call the nursing home just yet. Can all this slow down the aging process too?"

Once we approach and pass age forty, our environment (and that includes our nutrition) far surpasses heredity in health effects. So you can't blame Grandma for how *you* age, and *I* can't blame you. Antioxidants are an important link with protection against diseases associated with aging. Keep in mind that the accumulation of free radical damage increases with age.

No one can promise to turn the aging clock back for you, even though personal accounts of individual success stories are common. For many people, it seems as though the aging clock really can be made to run the other way. Of course, personal accounts are anecdotal evidence, and like a good researcher, I must discount these accounts as having no statistical significance. Then again, I've always firmly believed that anecdotal evidence is fine, *as long as I am the person in the anecdote!*

Antioxidants and food
Mom had one more question. Well, it was really her friend Jane's question, but it was one that kept coming up again and again: "Tell me why we can't get enough antioxidants from our regular food?"

We do get antioxidants in our fruits and vegetables, but only in very limited quantities. And like other healthful nutrients, the parts of food that contain them are often discarded – like fruit skins or the husks of grains.

Antioxidants are destroyed by cooking, storing, freezing, and canning. The antioxidant capacity of vegetables also decreases rapidly and significantly after most of them are taken apart or processed in any way. So foods are poor suppliers of antioxidants.

At the same time that we have greatly reduced access to natural antioxidants, our environmental and social factors conspire to place most of us in a very difficult – and dangerous – biochemical situation.

Since barely 9 percent of Americans eat the recommended five servings of fruits and vegetables per day, the opportunity for improving health by improving diet through nutraceutical supplementation is extremely critical. Although I encourage people to improve their food lifestyle, I know from clinical experience that a person would sooner give up his or her significant other than his or her diet habits. That's why I suggest nutraceuticals of the highest order available.

Here's another consideration: Dietary antioxidant levels in the blood show seasonal variations. DNA damage is lower in summer than in winter. And unless you have access to a local farmer's market, chances are your food, even in the summer, has traveled long distances – even all the way from other countries.

Dietary guidelines now recommended for the prevention of cancer are largely identical with those recommended for the prevention of cardiovascular disease. Indications are that oxidative damage contributes importantly to just about all degenerative diseases.

A final question
After a thoughtful moment of silent reflection, Mom asked: "Are my grandchildren taking nutraceuticals? Maybe young barley leaf powder?"

You better believe it, I replied. And so are your two great-grandchildren!

CHAPTER FIVE
THE POWER
OF GREEN

..in which we discuss chlorophyll, the greenish pigment found in plants – and learn just why it is so important.

SUN-KISSED

We often hear that ultraviolet light and exposure to the sun is harmful, causing everything from wrinkles to skin cancer. But didn't you ever wish you could package the wonderful *aura* that wraps around your entire being when you are lying in the sun? In a way, you do stow away some of the sun's benefits. Ultraviolet radiation causes a variety of biological effects that can be both positive and long lasting. Some examples:

~ Before surgery was used to treat bone degeneration, the sun was the recommended remedy.[1] Sunlight facilitates the construction of vitamin D in your skin, and your body is able to stockpile a supply during the summer to last you throughout the long, cold winter.[2] (Vitamin D is essential for bone mineralization. Its deficiency is recognized as a risk for hip fracture.[3])

~ A high percentage of adolescents, especially females, are at high risk of developing nutritional rickets, a disease marked by bending and distortion of bones. It's caused by vitamin D deficiency, especially in infancy and childhood. Longer exposure to the sun is a simple and effective preventive measure.[4]

~ Strange as it may sound, exposure to ultraviolet radiation can actually be cancer-*preventive*. (The strongest inverse correlations are with breast, colon, and ovarian cancers.)[5]

~ New mothers know all about the sun's benefits. Sunlight is the drug-free way of treating dry or cracked nipples, for getting rid of diaper rash, and for treating a new baby who is jaundiced.[6]

~ Dr. John Ott, photobiologist and pioneer in light research, discovered the benefits of natural light. His interest was piqued when his arthritis was apparently cured after breaking his eyeglasses while in Florida. He believed the effect of the direct ultraviolet light on his eyes was the critical factor. (Eyeglasses filter out a large percentage of ultraviolet rays, just as window glass does.)

A French physician noticed that his dog had an open sore on its back. Whenever he put a bandage on the area, the dog would rub it off on the fence post and go bask in the sun. Finally, the doctor let the dog be, and in a few days the sore healed. The doctor went on to develop "sun cures" for a variety of problems.

These are just a few of the potential positive things we are discovering about the effects of sunlight. Surely there are many other, as-yet-undiscovered health benefits streaming down upon us from that golden star at the center of our solar system.

In yet another way, the sun's goodness is being "bottled," and you don't have to sun bathe to reap the benefits. It all happens because of *chlorophyll*, the molecule that uses the sun's energy for sustaining the life of almost all green plants. (In general, plants cannot produce chlorophyll unless exposed to light.) Since we obtain our food by eating these plants (or by eating the animals that eat the plants), this process is said to be the source of human life as well. Let's find out why chlorophyll is so special.

"Chloro" is from the Greek *chloros*, which means yellowish green. The name of the element chlorine comes from the same source. (Chlorine is a yellowish green gas.) *Phyllum* means leaf.

> For those concerned about sun overexposure, recent studies demonstrate that botanical antioxidants can help protect against sun-induced damage. Antioxidants are even protective against melanoma (skin cancer). They can also reduce sun-mediated harm that has already occurred.[7]

FROM SEED TO SPROUT

From the time a seed germinates, it has one purpose in life: *to produce more seeds!* The process begins with a short blade of grass pushing itself above the soil to capture solar energy.

Once the grass makes its appearance, the leaves grow quickly, using sunlight as the basis for countless subsequent chemical processes that manufacture fats, amino acids, proteins, complex carbohydrates, and enzymes.

> The intricate machinations of this solar-powered factory in the leaves of the young grass plant are almost beyond comprehension.

But final results depend heavily on environmental factors. Without key nutrients from the soil and the right changes in climate, the sprouted seed misses the enzymes needed to enter the next growth phase.

Winter grasses grown in a greenhouse, although appearing to flourish, lack the nutrients necessary to develop into seed-bearing mature plants. The leaves cannot create the complicated organic molecules required for reproduction. It's like the difference between the eggs from the health store, which would have become chicks if fertilized, and the commercial eggs from the supermarket, which are far from fertile because of nutrient deficiencies. (You can even taste the difference!) Another example occurs at Thanksgiving. Virtually all mass-farmed turkeys have lost the ability to procreate. Without artificial insemination, they would vanish after a single generation. What's missing in these plants, in the eggs, and in the turkeys are a full profile of nutrients, as nature intended.

This is not to say that the sprouts you grow in your kitchen (without the benefit of soil) are not a valuable food. Because of their extreme freshness, I consider sprouts a vital part of my everyday diet. Sprouts are virtually the only food living and growing right up to the time they enter my mouth. They're also completely free of pesticides, additives, and other forms of food pollution – both intentional and incidental. So I'm not about to dismiss the importance of homegrown sprouts in the modern diet.

> Children particularly enjoy home sprouting because they can almost *see* the unborn, sleeping little stores of energy as the dormant seeds urge forward to life, slowly but surely.

FROM SPROUT TO GRAIN

The nutrients in the leaves of the young grass plant reach maximum concentration just before a phase in the plant's development called the *jointing stage*. This is when the stem begins to develop and chlorophyll, protein, and vitamin content decline, and fiber increases.[8]

So you can see why the young grass plant has a higher nutrient value than the grain. An amazing accumulation of nutrients found in barley grass are diminished in the grain. The greens are worth a king's ransom, as far as your health is concerned.

The sprouting process causes increased enzyme activity, an increase in protein, a decrease in starch, an increase in fiber, and higher amounts of certain vitamins and minerals. As carbohydrates decrease, the percentage of other nutrients increases.[9]

DO YOU HAVE THAT "GREEN" SHEEN?

Quietly, I play a game when I attend the major health food industry conventions. Before I know anything about the new people I meet, I try to guess what their diets are like. Of all the many dietary variations, I've found that there's only one that I can usually guess correctly: *the consumption of lots of green food or green supplements!* I note a kind of vibrancy in these people, a look of youth and energy reflected in skin tone and clear eyes. What I see is nothing that could be measured scientifically, but I'm convinced that it is there.

DEHYDRATION: THE BEST PRESERVATION PROCESS

Because it is so difficult to get a daily supply of fresh and organic green foods, supplementation is the alternative. Obviously, green foods transformed into supplements require some form of preservation. Dehydration is usually the method of choice.

Dehydrated foods evoke special memories for me. I can remember seeing strings suspended across my grandmother's kitchen ceiling every autumn. As a child, I stared wide-eyed at the apple pieces dangling from clothespins. The drying apple slices sent an aroma throughout the house, making our mouths water.

Grandma told us that the finished dried apples were not to be eaten now, but stashed away until the dead of winter. I did, however, manage to sneak a piece here and there when she wasn't looking. I wondered why the bits of dried apple were so much more pungent than fresh apples "in season."

Years later, I learned that the dried apples had higher values of concentrated nutrients, and thus a much more potent flavor.

On a portion-for-portion basis, dried foods have a significantly increased density of many nutrients, particularly the more stable minerals. Drying retains more nutritional value than toasting, roasting, steaming, baking or frying, mainly because the temperatures used are usually lower.

Because advanced technology has produced better drying chambers, this ancient method of food preservation is now in step with our 21st century lifestyle. We no longer have to hang fruit from our ceilings, and the finished product has higher nutrient retention than ever before.

Furthermore, dried foods make for easy availability – especially for supplementation. (Caution: Beware of sulfite-dried foods. They are destructive to our respiratory systems, and even life-threatening for asthmatics.)

> The advent of the supermarket is one of the worst things that ever happened to a vegetable. Dehydrated green foods lend a helping hand in our efforts to supersede that tragedy.

GREEN VEGETABLES AND THE GARBAGE STUDY

Several years ago, a team of researchers at a university in Chicago decided to treat the municipal dump as if it were an archaeological dig. The object was to scientifically evaluate food waste to see what inferences could be made about the eating habits of the society that produced the garbage.

The study makes fascinating reading for a number of reasons, but I mention it because of one important finding: A survey, with participants trying to accurately describe their own diets indicated that personal intake of green vegetables was *overestimated by a factor of three!*

So even if you *think* you eat a reasonable quantity of green vegetables, you are probably wrong. Want proof? Keep a record of everything you eat for two weeks. No cheating! Include the meals you had in restaurants and at parties. (Yes…they do count.) When you add the items in the fresh green veggie column, you may be disappointed.

Scientists generally concede that it is impossible to measure anything without creating change in some way, and this is a prime example of that phenomenon. If your two-week diary indicates substantial servings of green vegetables several times daily, it is very likely the result of the record keeping itself, so I'll still take credit, thank you. In other words, the quickest way to improve someone's diet is to ask them to write down everything they eat.

THE MAGIC OF CHLOROPHYLL

You don't need me to tell you to eat your greens. You can probably still hear your mother's voice scolding you with that same message. What's in vegetables that's so important? And why choose grasses instead of the more familiar dinner vegetables?

The answer takes us right back to chlorophyll, one of the main constituents that makes a green plant so valuable.

The fastest-growing plants have the most chlorophyll and the deepest green color. Cereal grasses grow the fastest!

Chlorophyll absorbs so strongly that it can mask the presence of other less powerful colors. When the chlorophyll molecule decays in the autumn, other more delicate colors are revealed. That's when we see the leaves turn red, orange, and golden brown (colors present because of molecules such as carotene and quercetin, explained in more depth later). Autumnal tints are a fascinating natural phenomenon, and the mechanism of chlorophyll breakdown in deciduous trees is still not fully understood.

Pigments reflect particular wavelengths of visible light, making them appear colorful. (The iris of your eye contains pigmented cells.) They are the means by which the energy of sunlight is captured for photosynthesis (explained on page 78). Since each pigment reacts with only a narrow range of the spectrum, there is usually a need to produce several kinds of pigments, each of a different color, to capture more of the sun's energy. And so the leaves are not only green, but also red, yellow, and orange.

Actually, chlorophyll absorbs light most strongly in the red and violet parts of the spectrum, the green light being very poorly absorbed. But when white light shines on chlorophyll-containing structures such as plant leaves, green light is transmitted and reflected, and the structures appear green.

A LITTLE BIOCHEMISTRY

We breathe because the process of converting carbohydrates into energy consumes oxygen. All animal cells using energy require oxygen when they burn carbohydrates, giving off carbon dioxide as a product of this reaction. This process is called *respiration*. It's not unlike burning a log in the fireplace, in terms of what goes in and what comes out.

Green plants, on the other hand, use *solar* energy.

> Green plants actually *make* carbohydrates from nothing more than sunlight, water, and carbon dioxide – creating organic substances from inorganic chemicals, converting the energy from the sun into chemical energy.

The plant's roots gather the water, and the carbon dioxide is collected from the air around pores that are under the leaves. That process is called *photosynthesis* and chlorophyll is the chemical that makes it possible.

So without chlorophyll, the plant couldn't take carbon dioxide and water and do its magic. *With chlorophyll, it transforms these lifeless substances into food.*

No wonder chlorophyll is known as "concentrated sunlight." The chemical energy stored by photosynthesis in carbohydrates drives biochemical reactions in nearly all living organisms.

> When the plant changes the water and carbon dioxide into glucose, it releases oxygen into the air. The plant mixes the sugar with water and sends it to other parts of the plant to be used as food.

GREEN "BLOOD"

An intriguing fact about chlorophyll is its similarity to hemoglobin, the molecule that transports oxygen in your own blood. Hemoglobin and chlorophyll share a structure called the *porphyrin ring*. In hemoglobin, there's an iron atom bonded inside the ring; but chlorophyll has a magnesium atom there instead.

Because chlorophyll's magnesium atom is replaced by hydrogen ions in cooking, chlorophyll is easily damaged by heat. This changes the molecular structure, causing alterations that make cooked green vegetables paler in color.

It is tempting to speculate whether chlorophyll in food can be used to help manufacture new blood cells in our bodies. For more than a century, ever since the green pigment in plants was identified and called chlorophyll, scientists have puzzled over this question. It was early in the last century that the similarity between hemoglobin and chlorophyll was confirmed.

Extra energy comes from extra red blood cells carrying oxygen to our cells. Because chlorophyll and hemoglobin are nearly identical in structure, with only the difference of the one atom at their center, it has been theorized that enzymes in our blood easily convert chlorophyll into hemoglobin.

Although chlorophyll-rich plants contain nutrients that have been shown to be important for healthy blood, the *direct* use of the chlorophyll molecule has yet to be scientifically demonstrated.

Yoshide Hagiwara, MD, in his book *Green Barley Essence: The Ideal Fast Food,* suggests a mechanism whereby chlorophyll may stimulate the production of hemoglobin by an indirect route. Although the intact chlorophyll molecule is difficult to absorb, there is a ring-opening process that facilitates this assimilation.

The parts of the chlorophyll molecule are reassembled later as hemoglobin, with iron substituted for magnesium.

"Thus, the conclusion drawn from my reasoning," writes Dr. Hagiwara, "is that the green blood of the plant can become the red blood of man."[10]

The best way to get chlorophyll in your diet is to eat organic dark green leafy vegetables, freshly picked.

Did I hear you groan? Second best is to eat carefully prepared special products made from these plants, designed to preserve the chlorophyll. A select few can be convenient, easy, reliable, and healthful.

You may be saying: "But I have a salad every day. Isn't that enough?"

No! Most salads, at least most salads as eaten in North America, are comprised of head (or iceberg) lettuce. Head lettuce is a worthless vegetable on the table, and compared to green lettuce varieties, it looks like a junk food.

"What?" you respond. "Lettuce a junk food? Explain this!"

For starters, lettuce is mostly water. Okay, no big deal. But it's also very low in the all-important chlorophyll because the head construction prevents sunlight from being harnessed and reaching most of the leaves. Makes sense — there's no reason for the plant to have chlorophyll in its leaves if there's little light for photosynthesis.

But head lettuce has been genetically engineered almost beyond cellular recognition. Grown with large amounts of pesticides and sprays to preserve crispness, it's groomed so it won't look "tired."

HEMOGLOBIN

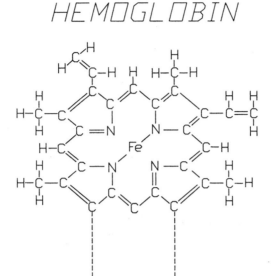

Fe = Iron

CHLOROPHYLL

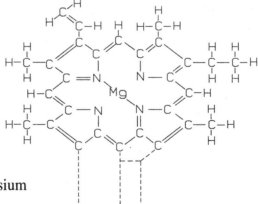

Mg = Magnesium

Note the similarity between our hemoglobin molecule and the plant's chlorophyll
molecule.

After all, it has a long journey to restaurants and supermarkets across the country. With nutrients absent and toxins present, if iceberg lettuce appears fresh, it's only an illusion.

Iceberg lettuce should go the way of the marshmallows that used to be so popular in fruit salad. Let the food industry work a little harder in our behalf.

Sure, you could get organic head lettuce. But why not use butterhead (Boston and Bibb), Cos (romaine), leaf lettuce, or even spinach, kale, or any one of a dozen tastier and more nutritious alternatives?

Having chosen a healthful salad variety, you also have to be careful with the salad dressing. Watch out for products containing polyunsaturated vegetable oils.

> **Oil in salad dressing is almost guaranteed to be at least partially oxidized or rancid as a result of processing, storage, and exposure to heat, light, and air.**

What's more, your body might take advantage of the quick energy fix from the oil, carbohydrate, or sugar in the salad dressing and fail to fully utilize the green stuff. (We have found one delightful exception, *grapeseed oil*, which is the most stable of all oils available.)

Will you have a salad left after you banish the head lettuce and the dressing? If you do, you might have some good stuff in your salad bowl. Fresh carrots, for example. But are they thin-sliced or shredded? And how long have they been like that, exposed to the air? This goes for the cucumbers and green peppers. The very process of preparing a salad takes time, leaving the vegetables unprotected and exposed to air and light in potentially deleterious ways.

With minor exceptions, the more thinly the veggies are sliced, the more quickly oxidation erodes their vitamins and enzymes. (Minerals are pretty safe here.) By the time they get from the big farm to the supermarket to your grocery bag to your refrigerator to your table, they're already considerably degraded. Go heavy on sprouts and leafy greens in that salad because they don't have to be mushed, mashed, or mangled before you serve them.

> Fortunately, most vegetables have a wonderfully complex and "smart" skin structure that keeps air and pathogens from "breaking and entering."

CHLOROPHYLL FOR ATHLETES

Chlorophyll has been called the "Green Steroid" because of its positive effects on muscle endurance. Green foods promote anabolic processes, the chemical reactions that *build* and *repair* tissue. On the other hand, catabolic actions *consume* tissue for energy. In cases of extreme physical performance (such as when an athlete is pushed to the limit of endurance), it's the catabolic process that causes fatigue and tissue breakdown.

Remember a ship named the *Henrietta*? It was featured in Jules Verne's *Around the World in Eighty Days*. Running low on fuel in the middle of the ocean, the crew burned the entire superstructure in the boiler to keep on steaming ahead. The voyage was completed on schedule, but the ship looked more like an empty barge than a passenger ship when it arrived at its destination.

I think of the *Henrietta* whenever I see an athlete at the limit of exhaustion. He may be winning the race, but he's burning up his body to do it. A good supply of chlorophyll can delay that decisive moment – the moment of exhaustion.

INDOOR EDENS: GREEN LEAVES AND POLLUTED INDOOR ENVIRONMENTS

Because plants emit oxygen, they have been used indoors for purifying "bad" air for more than two hundred years. Early experiments demonstrated this phenomenon by "clearing the air" after burning candles (when candles were used extensively prior to the discovery of electricity).

Different parts of the leaf have different jobs. The veins in a leaf are bundles of tiny tubes that carry water and minerals to the leaf and return food from the leaf to the rest of the plant. On the underside of the leaf are small openings or pores, which serve as the lungs of the leaf, allowing air to enter. These openings allow the evaporation of water and the release of oxygen – just what we need in a stuffy, polluted environment. (Chances are your bedroom TV contributes to the pollution.) Now you might look twice at that wilting ficus in every doctor's waiting room!

THE HEALING POWER OF CHLOROPHYLL

Chlorophyll has strong antibacterial action, and clears up odors of putrefaction effectively. It has been used in surgery, in ulcerative carcinoma, in head colds, acute rhinitis (inflammation of mucus membranes of the nose), and chronic ear infections and inflammations. It has also been used for diabetic leg ulcers, contagious impetigo (a scabby, pustular skin eruption), rectal sores, vaginitis, and infection of the uterine cervix.

~ Chlorophyll, the perfect host for magnesium, is helpful in protecting against muscle cramping, menstrual problems, menopausal symptoms, cardiovascular disease, bronchial spasms, and anemia.

~ Chlorophyll is an example of a plant compound that can protect DNA from damage caused by chemical or physical agents.[11]

~ Its nucleic and amino acid profiles meet the protein needs of our brain because these help to build neuropeptides.

~ Chlorophyll served as both disinfectant and antibiotic during the Civil War. Today we use it to treat sewage waste.

~ A study using chlorophyll derivatives showed that chlorophyll contains an antimutagenic agent, effective against many carcinogens.[12]

~ Food sources that yield chlorophyll derivatives may play a significant role in cancer prevention.[13]

Regarded as one of the most powerful healers on earth, humans ate greens for three million years, long before we first made tools or discovered fire.

Many healthcare providers, involved in the alternative medicine movement, confirm that blended greens, powdered greens, or juiced greens are the secret to healing. For the last twenty-five years, I have personally witnessed the healing process of countless numbers of people at special health facilities. Most of these people had very serious degenerative diseases, and many had been given up by the traditional medical community. A program of *greens* helped to turn things around.

Since too many of us cannot afford to visit these places long enough to heal, green nutraceuticals can function as amazing elixirs. Don't wait for the "human condition" – the diseased state that wears you down, reduces quality of life, and shortens lifespan. If chlorophyll is therapeutic, it is no doubt also preventive. So take it *before* you need it.

CHAPTER SIX
KNOW YOUR NUTRIENTS

...in which we discuss and explain substances such as enzymes, flavonoids, vitamins, and minerals — why they are so important to your health, and why greens are your best source.

LEAVE THE PYRAMIDS TO THE PHARAOHS

Whether right side up or upside down, those commonly seen food pyramids have yet to demonstrate that they serve any useful purpose when it comes to getting us to change the way we eat. These six words, simplistic as they may seem, may be the best guideline possible: ***high* plant intake = *low* disease incidence.**

We have only recently learned that there is much more to nutrition than just the consumption of vitamins and minerals. Even learning about the exceptional nutrients found in plant foods – and even knowing which plants are teeming with these particular nutrients – may still not be inspiration enough for you to alter your eating habits. The odds are better that such information will help you to select a choice easy-to-swallow nutraceutical – especially when you learn that such a product can fill in the nutritional blanks your body requires for optimum health *with very little effort.*

In addition to chlorophyll, many plant foods contain phytochemicals associated with protection from – and treatment of – heart disease, diabetes, hypertension, cancer, and an array of other degenerative diseases.

> But you claim the benefits only when the levels of these individual phytonutrients reach beyond those you get from your normal balanced diet.[1]

We already know that a broad class of phytochemicals is ubiquitous in the plant kingdom. Because their health-protective properties are dependent on their *cumulative* impact, you want to be sure that your nutraceutical preference includes most, if not all, of the substances described in detail in this chapter.

> Preventive substances found in plants may inhibit carcinogen activation, enhance carcinogen detoxification, prevent carcinogens from interacting with critical target sites in the body, and impede tumor progression.

A description of some of the most significant plant phytochemicals follows.

NEW FRIENDS: NUTRIENTS NOT WELL-KNOWN

Superoxide Dismutase (SOD)

I can remember when researchers struggled to define the word enzyme, when the scientific jargon was ahead of a clear definition. We knew that enzymes were important, but we didn't always know why.

After further study, scientists learned that an enzyme was a complex protein produced by living cells, acting as a catalyst for specific biochemical reactions. And the deeper they were studied, the more the function and importance of enzymes became understood. It appeared that nothing of consequence occurred in your body without this or that particular enzyme sparking the action.

We can hardly pick up a medical journal or a bottle of multinutrient supplements without seeing the word enzyme. The journals extol their benefits, providing intricate explanations of how the various pathways work.

The nutrient companies add cofactors to assist the absorption process. The effectiveness of enzymes in general, however, is still considered superior when they are ingested as part of a whole food, or as found in whole-food supplements.

Eventually, we learned about a few enzymes that were infinitely superior, inclduing SOD. This enzyme protects against oxidant-induced damage, functioning as a potent scavenger of free radicals. It has the capability of preventing fats from changing into harmful lipid peroxide (the toxic form). It also has anti-inflammatory properties and it is easily digested.

> Peroxides and superoxides are free radicals. *Glutathione peroxidase* and *superoxide dismutase* are enzymes that reduce these toxins. These enzymes are especially important when you eat fried foods, which have an excess of oxidized fat byproducts (the reason these foods are so damaging to your health).

Because SOD is so remarkable, manufacturers began to detach it from its food source and to encapsulate it. Whether or not SOD is useful this way is still a highly controversial topic. Taken orally, in isolated form, its benefits are questionable.[2]

Since free radical damage is the hallmark of aging, and since SOD is a free radical scavenger, it is considered an anti-aging nutrient. Studies validate that it is protective against cancer, arthritis, radiation exposure, and the inflammatory aspects of cardiovascular disease, among other problems. Here are results of some of the research:.

~ *Exercise.* We all know about the benefits of exercise. One of its advantages is that exercising decreases the level of the free radical, superoxide. It does this by increasing SOD activity in the aorta and heart.[3]

~ *Cancer.* SOD may send signals that interfere with the damage caused by oxidative stress, especially in tumor tissues. For this reason SOD is considered crucial in affecting the survival of cancer patients. Levels of SOD can even serve as an indication of prognosis for certain kinds of cancer.[4]

~ *Parkinson's disease.* Since oxidative stress reactions may contribute to this disease, SOD plays a significant role by detoxifying the superoxide radical.[5]

~ *Preterm infant lung disease.* Free oxygen radicals have been implicated in lung disease in preterm infants. SOD for the pregnant mother provides a defense against such oxidant injury.[6]

~ *Aging.* Treatment with SOD increased the average lifespan of test animals by 44 percent. When given to prematurely aging animals, the result increase lifespan by 67 percent.[7] Deficiencies in SOD also strongly shortened the lifespan of yeast cells. These studies confirm the involvement of free radicals in human aging.[8]

~ *Rheumatoid arthritis.* Very low levels of circulating SOD are observed in those with rheumatoid arthritis, and these levels significantly improve when SOD is added to their treatment, ultimately reducing symptoms.[9]

~ *Asthma.* Loss of SOD activity occurs within minutes of an acute asthmatic response. This decreased activity contributes to airway inflammation and injury through increased formation of toxic free radicals, and suggests that enrichment of lung antioxidants is therapeutic for asthma.[10]

~ *Ischemia.* Disturbance in oxidant-antioxidant balance renders heart tissue more vulnerable to free radical injuries. In the presence of ischemia, SOD activities decrease significantly.[11] (Ischemia is a condition of low oxygen, usually due to obstruction of the arterial blood supply or inadequate blood flow.)

~ *Sclerosis.* Administration of SOD may be effective in the therapeutic approach in systemic sclerosis.[12]

~ *Gingivitis.* SOD can reduce free radical damage to gingival
tissues, helping to maintain oral health.[13]

You can see that SOD plays an essential protective role against
free radical tissue damage observed in inflammatory states.[14] This
may be a key factor in its ability to alleviate some of the conditions outlined above.

Enzymes are not present in cooked food because they are destroyed at 118° F (47° C). For proper function, enzymes also require the presence of adequate coenzymes, vitamins, minerals,
and electrolytes.

Many people with digestive disorders find relief taking SOD before meals. The best source is obviously raw foods – one reason
why young cereal grass sprouts are excellent nutraceuticals.
(Young barley leaf powder has a high SOD content.) SOD stops
the damage caused by free radicals by converting them to harm-
less molecules of oxygen and water.

Carotenes

Carotenoids are usually the major pigments in flowers and fruits,
with colors ranging from red to yellow. The red of a ripe tomato
is produced by its carotenoids. So is the orange of a carrot, and
that particular carotenoid is called *carotene* – which is the precursor of vitamin A. (For the biochemists among you, each molecule of carotene gives rise to two vitamin A molecules.)

As explained, carotenoids are usually masked by chlorophyll. In
the autumn, as the quantity of chlorophyll in the leaf declines,
the carotenoids become visible and this produces the vibrant yel-
lows, oranges, and reds of autumn foliage.

Color on the Dinner Plate

Red foods contain lycopene, the pigment in tomatoes, which are localized in the prostate gland

Yellow-green vegetables, such as corn and leafy greens, contain lutein and zeaxanthin, which are localized in the retina

Red-purple foods contain anthocyannins, found in apples, grapes, berries, and wine

Orange foods contain carotene, and include carrots, mangos, apricots, pumpkin and winter squash

Orange-yellow foods contain flavonoids, and include oranges, tangerines, and lemons

Green foods contain glucosinolates, and include broccoli, brussel sprouts, and kale

White-green foods contain allyl sulfides, found in the onion family

We are advised to ingest one serving of each of these groups daily. Do you think you could incorporate this advice in your daily food selections?

You are no doubt familiar with beta-carotene. Did you know that there are at least twelve different carotenes? And did you know that alpha-carotene might be more important than the beta form? If you eat a carrot, or drink a young barley leaf powder mix, you get all twelve of the carotene factions (and probably a few more that have yet to be identified).

If you take a beta-carotene supplement, you get only the beta component, and it may not be the one you need most. When studies are done to evaluate the protection observed with carotenoid-rich vegetable juices, beta-carotene accounts for only part of the positive results.[15]

The reason that beta-carotene had become a more familiar word, while alpha was virtually unknown, is very simple: beta-carotene is easier to synthesize commercially. So naturally this is the form that has been promoted and sold.

> Body cells can convert carotenes to vitamin A as required, provided we are in good health. The carotene in leafy greens is converted to vitamin A about twice as efficiently as the carotene in carrots and other root vegetables.[16]

Alpha-carotene is far more effective than beta-carotene in combating some types of human cancer cells. A report in the *Journal of the National Cancer Institute* states: "We found that natural carotene extracted from palm oil suppresses the proliferation of various human malignant tumor cells. . . . It was about ten times more inhibitory than beta-carotene."[17]

This is yet another good argument for obtaining most of your nutrients from food or nutrient-dense food supplements – sources that are far more likely to contain the full range of carotenes – as opposed to synthetic extractions.

The reason carotenes are such effective antioxidants is related to the process of photosynthesis, described in chapter 5. Plants that convert solar energy to chemical energy must deal with an immense number of charged particles. The sun's rays, in the form of photons, send electrons bouncing in every direction. With the aid of chlorophyll (and hundreds of other chemicals) the result is the manufacture of carbohydrates and the release of oxygen.

One would think that this reaction, going on right there inside the plant leaf cells, would be extremely damaging to the surrounding cells. These cells do require powerful protection from the onslaught of stray charges, and they get it from *carotenes*. That explains why the darkest, greenest plants – the ones with the most chlorophyll – tend to have such high concentrations of carotenes. In general, the darker the green vegetable, the higher the carotene concentration. Where there is lots of chlorophyll there is also plenty of carotene.

Here are some recent studies validating the benefits of carotenes:

~ Carotenoids, including carotenes, are potentially useful chemopreventive agents. (*Journal of Nutrition*[18])

~ Carotenes have photoprotective effects in your skin, efficiently scavenging radicals and inhibiting harmful lipid peroxidation (rancidity). Taking too much carotene, however, can lead to pro-oxidant effects, rather than antioxidant benefits. (*Photochemical Photobiology*[19]) That's a risk associated with carotenes when consumed in isolated form. This does not happen when the carotenes are part of a food complex, when the amount ingested would be naturally self-limiting.

~ There is a correlation between the antioxidant activity of leaf pigments and the carotenoid content in the leaf. (*Phytochemistry Analysis*[20])

~ Carotenes can help your body to utilize vitamin C. They appear to have the ability to inhibit the activity of inflammation-causing enzymes.

~ Vegetable carotenoids have a protective role in the macular region of the retina, thereby helping to prevent macular degeneration. (*Journal of Nutrition*[21])

~ Leafy greens rich in carotenoids might have the potential to reduce the risk of prostate cancer. (*Journal of Nutrition*[22])

~ Increased concentrations of carotenoids have been associated with a decreased risk of degenerative diseases. (*Journal of Nutrition*[23])

Catechins

Cancer chemoprevention is a new and important medical science and much interest has been focused on catechins, not only for their antioxidant activity, but also because they help to prevent the formation of tumors or cell mutations.[24]

Catechins belong to a family of substances called flavonoids. Flavonoids are found in a wide variety of plant products, such as fruit, vegetables, herbs, nuts, and tea, and have a broad range of beneficial effects, including protection from cardiovascular disease and certain forms of cancer. Flavonoids are a group of more than 4,000 polyphenolic antioxidants, and catechins are one of the six major groups of flavonoids.[25]

> The more flavonoids you consume, the less chance you have of being at risk for coronary artery disease and cancer.[26]

The high antioxidant activity of flavonoids contributes to their beneficial effects.[27] But catechins, which are produced by the metabolism of the flavonoids, are even more powerful than the flavonoids from which they are derived. (Such substances are called *metabolites*, so catechins are metabolites of flavonoids.)

Surely you've heard of the benefits of green tea. Well, it's the catechin content of the green leaves in green tea that is known to have antiviral properties.[28] They also reduce inflammation in individuals with inflammatory arthritis. Catechins accomplish this through their ability to inhibit the breakdown of proteoglycan and type II collagen – thereby slowing down cartilage destruction. Proteoglycans and type II collagen are substances essential for healthy joint function.

For detailed information on these nutrients and their arthritis connection, refer to my book *The Remarkable Healing Power of Velvet Antler.*[29]

Because catechins can suppress lipid peroxidation and increase enzyme activity, they appear capable of protecting the liver against toxic invasion.[30] Research also shows that certain catechins might be potent neuroprotective agents against Parkinson's disease.[31]

Catechins, whether from tea or other sources, may reduce the risk of ischemic heart disease mortality, but not of stroke.[32]

> The natural abundance and favorable bioavailability of catechins make them a promising addition to the list of potential colorectal cancer preventive agents.[33]

An extensive study done in the Netherlands showed that people who consumed the least amount of green leaves (usually from tea) showed a higher risk of aortic atherosclerosis.[34]

Most of the studies performed to date on flavonoids and some of their metabolites (in this case, the catechins) used forms present in foods. As summed up in the *European Journal of Clinical Nutrition*:

> "Catechins are quantitatively important bioactive components of the daily diet, which should be taken into account when studying the relation between diet and chronic diseases."[35]

OLD FRIENDS:
BETTER KNOWN NUTRIENTS

No chapter on nutrients would be complete without mentioning those with which we are already quite familiar. Although by no means a complete compendium, the nutrients discussed here are those found in significant quantities in leafy greens.

Vitamins

Vitamin C

If I had been in charge of naming the vitamins, I would have named vitamin C *first* and called it vitamin A. Vitamin C is necessary for *any* biological process requiring nutrients to pass through cell membranes – and that includes just about *all* metabolic actions we know about. Perhaps the most important role of vitamin C is to help prevent the proteins in the cell membranes from being damaged by oxidation.

Proteins are large, complex, and specialized molecules that control the functioning of cell membranes. They let nutrients in, send waste products out, and block entry to toxic or viral invaders. Cell membrane proteins are responsible for immune responses on the cellular level, *where it really counts*. When a protein is oxidized, it's split apart and destroyed.

> **Vitamin C works by rushing in first and neutralizing the free radicals before they can do their damage to cell membranes and other tissues. That's why it's recognized as a powerful antioxidant.**

Interestingly, humans and a few other primates (apes and chimpanzees) are the only mammals that don't synthesize their own vitamin C.[36] We have three of the four necessary enzymes, and it's speculated that we lost the fourth (L-gulonolactone oxidase) through evolutionary misfortune. Not a huge problem if you're living in the woods and eating everything fresh off the vine. In fact, that's probably why we have a "sweet tooth" – our body is seeking out the freshest, most vitamin-rich fruits and greens (often very sweet tasting). But put that same primate in the convenience store instead of the jungle, and you get a different result: lots of sugar, no vitamins, and degenerating health.

The missing enzyme is necessary for the last step in the transfer of sugar to ascorbic acid. Again, no problem if you eat fruits and vegetables with high ascorbate content. Too bad we can't make vitamin C from sugar, as other animals do. Actually, most commercially manufactured ascorbates are made from glucose!

The best way to get vitamin C is from food. Bioflavonoids, associated with vitamin C in nature, are still not fully understood. Synthetic ascorbic acid, chemically similar to vitamin C (or *almost* similar – sometimes it's a molecular "mirror image") lacks cofactors like bioflavonoids. A complete plant leaf is guaranteed to have all these cofactors.

> Because there's so much we don't know about how vitamins work, the best source of vitamins will always be the whole foods that contain them – not necessarily because the vitamins themselves are any different, but because other substances, commonly found with the vitamins, have important but as yet unidentified roles to play.

Vitamin A

About ten million children the world over are deficient in vitamin A. Over one million suffer from varying degrees of visual impairment every year due to this deficiency.

"This problem is likely to be seriously magnified [in a few years]," reads a report in the *Journal of Ophthalmic Nursing Technology*. "The scope of the problem is immense, and the need to address it is urgent, representing one of the greatest failures in global public health planning," conclude the researchers, who suggest that vitamin A deficiency could be eradicated with *vegetables*.[37]

While most of the vitamin A deficiency problems exist in third world countries, the effects are seen here in the US as well.

Much of the research cited earlier links vitamin A intake to cancer resistance. Patrick Quillin sums it up perfectly in his book *Healing Nutrients*: "So important is vitamin A in preventing cancer that serum levels of vitamin A are like a crystal ball in predicting who will get cancer: the lower the level of serum vitamin A (and/or carotene) the greater the risk for cancer."[38]

> It's not difficult to be vitamin A deficient. Antagonists to this nutrient include air pollutants, exposure to glare or strong light, nitrate fertilizers, vitamin D deficiency, alcohol, coffee, cortisone, and mineral oil.

As with vitamin E, concentrations of vitamin A are lower in those with Alzheimer's disease than in those not afflicted.[39] The list of benefits of this nutrient is extensive, and the harmful consequences of deficiency are of major concern worldwide. Only at *extremes* of deficiency does your blood show a vitamin A deficiency – and no one is likely to take samples of their liver to check the status. Vitamin A deficiency is also associated with periodontal disease.[40]

Zinc deficiency interferes with the absorption of vitamin A, and because zinc and vitamin A deficiency often coexist, simultaneous zinc and vitamin A intake (or consumption of nutraceuticals containing both) may help to improve vitamin A deficiency.[41]

Because vitamin A is a fat-soluble vitamin – which means it gets stored in your body, rather than released like the B and C vitamins – toxicity can be a problem when it is ingested in supplemental form. Although deficiency is observed in some precancerous conditions, and can adversely affect your immune system, an excess of this nutrient can also be harmful.[42]

More than 72,000 registered nurses from eleven states, aged thirty-four to seventy-seven, were studied over a period of eighteen years. Women with the highest vitamin A intake had a significantly elevated relative risk of hip fracture compared with women with the smallest intake (less than 1,250 micrograms a day).[43]

> The fact that elevated levels of harmful substances occur after supplementation with excess amounts of vitamin A, but not after eating liver (a rich source of vitamin A), strongly argues our key point: Get it from food, not from isolated supplements![44]

The B Vitamins
If you're on *antibiotics* or take aspirin or other drugs; if you happen to be *fasting* because your friend said it would make you feel great; if, like most of the world, you're *dieting*; if you're under *stress* because of a traffic jam, deadline, or mother-in-law problems; or if, like just about all of us, a major portion of your food is *cooked* (have I missed anyone?), more than likely you are vitamin B deficient!

Because they are water-soluble, B vitamins are not usually stored in your body, so it isn't difficult to suffer short-term deficiencies, especially since most B vitamins are easily damaged or destroyed by the cooking process. Some are produced by intestinal bacteria, but be aware that if you're taking antibiotics, your normal supply of beneficial bacteria may be cut off. (Antibiotics are not selective; they annihilate all bacteria, including the "good-guy" flora.)

Although B vitamins are usually bundled together in foods, each separate type can have a very distinct function. Some play a major role in amino acid and enzyme production. Others participate in immune function and the regulation of certain toxins. B_6, for example, works to prevent an amino acid from damaging arterial walls that causes atherosclerosis and coronary disease later on. For this reason, B_6 deficiency may be a major factor in heart disease, the number one killer in the US.

Folic acid (another B vitamin, named for the foliage in which it is found) helps to regulate new cell growth and is related to immune responses.

B vitamins are also linked to proper functioning and health of the nervous system, skin, hair, and eyes. B_6 deficiencies are linked to arthritis; folic acid to anemia; B_6 and B_{12} to carpal tunnel syndrome; B_6 with PMS; and niacin (B_3) with high cholesterol and insulin intolerance.

Vitamins B_1 (thiamine) and B_2 (riboflavin) are two very important B vitamins whose significance is often overshadowed by the others. Until recently, thiamine deficiency has been considered to be mainly the result of alcoholism. We know better now.

Despite its importance, thiamine can be harmful if taken in supplemental form.

When we check ingredient listings on food packages, we are usually pleased to see nutrient additions. Thiamine is commonly added to basic foods such as milled flour, cereals, peanut butter, refreshment drinks, and pastas. Beware! Used this way, the thiamine supplementation may enhance cancer rates.[45] Another demonstration of the importance of getting our nutrients from whole foods. The enzyme that helps to degrade excess thiamine is found in raw and fermented fish and in certain vegetables (barley leaf).

Thiamine deficiency, more common than generally realized, is also associated with cognitive impairment.[46] This nutrient acts as a special kind of antioxidant, and its deficiency leads to neurodegeneration.[47] Serious symptoms can result from a continual low intake of thiamine, including feelings of anxiety. In addition to losses in cooking, baking powder and soda also destroy thiamine in muffins, breads, and cakes.

Riboflavin also has a long list of benefits, but what stands out is its relationship to homocysteine (that unwanted stuff that affects our hearts). We keep hearing about folic acid, B_6, and B_{12} to lower homocysteine levels. Well, guess what! Riboflavin deficiency is also correlated with high homocysteine levels.[48]

Because exercise stresses the pathways that depend on thiamine and riboflavin, the requirements for these vitamins may be increased in athletes and active individuals.[49] Unfortunately, signs of marginal B vitamin deficiencies are difficult to detect.

Young barley leaves supply generous amounts of both B1 and B2.

Vitamin D
Vitamin D is one vitamin you don't necessarily need to ingest – you can synthesize it yourself from exposure to sunlight. When skin is exposed to the ultraviolet rays of the sun, a precursor of vitamin D is manufactured from a form of cholesterol (one of many important functions of cholesterol). This substance is then converted into the active form of vitamin D by your liver and kidneys.

Vitamin D is important in regulating both the calcium and phosphorous flow into and out of bone structure, as well as for numerous other functions related to your heart, nervous system, and blood. Because it is produced in one part of your body (skin) and has a controlling effect on other tissues (bone), vitamin D can be thought of as more hormone-like than vitamin-like. The converted form of vitamin D (1-25-dihydroxycholecalciferol) is closely related chemically to estrogen and cortisone.

Unfortunately, the practice of regular sunbathing has been drastically curtailed by the prevailing "wisdom" that sunlight is bad for you. Nothing could be farther from the truth!

Skin cancer is more common than ovarian, cervical, central nervous system cancer, or leukemia. Melanoma (skin cancer) is increasing faster than any other cancer in the United States, as well as all over the world. "And you're still going to say it's okay to sunbathe?" I hear you ask, incredulously. Well, think about this trend again. Certainly Americans are not spending any more time in the sun than they did a generation ago. In fact, just the opposite is true. We are more likely to spend time in the glow of the TV set. As a nation, our lifestyle has become ever more sedentary – enclosed in buildings and protected from the sun.

If the correlation between sun exposure and malignant skin cancer were that simple, surely skin cancer rates would be dropping!

Note the following research:

~ *International Journal of Epidemiology*: Lack of exposure to ultraviolet sunlight can increase the prevalence of vitamin D deficiency and may place some women at higher risk of breast cancer. A significant negative association was found between breast cancer incidence and total sunlight levels.[50]

~ *Preventive Medicine*: Regular sunning could prevent far more breast cancer fatalities than the skin cancer fatalities it would cause.[51]

~ *Cancer*: Ultraviolet radiation may protect against clinical prostate cancer.[52]

~ *Anticancer Research*: Mortality rates from prostate cancer in the United States are inversely correlated with ultraviolet radiation, the principal source of vitamin D.[53]

Still want to hide from the sun? Not me! On the other hand, the risk of damaging your skin is very real.

The increase of serious skin cancer should not be ignored just because other life-threatening risks may be reduced.

While vitamin D may explain part of the beneficial effect of sunlight, we still need to understand what is failing in our skin that makes us so much more susceptible to skin cancer than our ancestors were just a few generations ago.

The answer? Antioxidants, which are themselves easily oxidized because of their "sacrificial" role, intercepting reactive particles (free radicals) before they damage vital lipids and proteins. Not only is skin exposed directly to the mutagenic solar radiation, but skin also has a very high rate of regeneration for healing wounds and for replacing worn-out tissue.

Viewed on a small enough scale, it's correct to say that everyone always has skin cancer. The DNA in skin cells is constantly subjected to damage from high-energy sunlight. When this happens, the cell's "programming" to regenerate sometimes takes over. Uncontrolled cell proliferation, fortunately, is the exception rather than the rule. Cells can communicate with each other via an astoundingly complex chemical language, and the programs in the undamaged DNA can identify abnormal cell propagation and shut down the new cell line. So in the presence of enough antioxidants, your smart body knows how to protect you from sun exposure.

One interesting study of melanoma in Moscow concluded that consumption of greens significantly decreased the risk of this disease.[54]

This is certainly not a surprising result, and it suggests that the real problem with sunlight and skin cancer is *nutritional*. Keep your skin (and body!) well supplied with antioxidants and the risk is minimized.

> It cannot be overemphasized that the best natural sources of antioxidants are the greenest and fastest-growing plants.

This makes sense in light of what we learned earlier about what goes on inside the leaf of a plant. Extremely high-energy solar radiation is being used to drive the photosynthesis reaction, which in some ways is the reverse of oxidation. It's critical to keep the newly formed products of the plant – the carbohydrates and free oxygen – from bouncing right back in the other direction. It's also important to control the unwanted effects of all that high-energy radiation and those highly charged particles associated with the photosynthesis process.

New material is being synthesized at a phenomenal rate as the plant grows. Again, with such powerful electrical and chemical forces at work, a large supply of antioxidants is necessary to keep these processes from causing major damage.

Of course you should be careful not to overdo sunbathing; burning your skin is not good for you. But a healthy tan is exactly that – *healthy*!

Someday soon, the high priests of medical wisdom will understand how important sunshine is to our health.

> The implication for sun worshipers is clear: eat lots of fresh green plants, with an emphasis on the young sprouted shoots.

Vitamin D deficiency is the most common nutritional deficiency in Crohn's disease, which is fast replacing ulcers as one of the more common digestive disorders among Americans. It is interesting to note that glass, clothing, and smog block the ultraviolet rays that create vitamin D, but clouds do not. So the healthy effects of sunlight are available even on hazy or overcast days.

Vitamin E

Vitamin E has been credited with everything from improved sex hormone production to prevention of hair loss. We do know that vitamin E, another fat-soluble antioxidant, offers protection against heart and vascular disease and against a wide range of toxic substances.

One problem with vitamin E supplements, however, is that the oil-based products from which they are extracted are usually very unstable. Light, heat, air, and age render the oil rancid and the value of the supplement questionable. What this means is that we should not rely completely on supplemental forms of vitamin E. As usual, it's much better to get it from food. And where do we find vitamin E? In whole grains, eggs, avocados, sweet potatoes, asparagus, broccoli – and, you guessed it: *green leafy vegetables.*

Vitamin E deficiency is associated with the kind of diet that raises your cholesterol, and its deficiency also exacerbates lipid peroxidation.

The beneficial effects of vitamin E are due to its powerful antioxidant actions.[55] We've known about the value of vitamin E for fertility and for reducing menopausal symptoms for years. Newer studies show that vitamin E:

~ can reduce health problems caused by exposure to second-hand smoke[56]

~ assists in enhancing sexual function because it is essential for the release of estrogen from cells, improves the activity of nitric oxide, and plays an important role in the signaling aspects of smooth muscle cells[57]

~ helps to lower homocysteine levels[58]

~ seems to uncouple joint inflammation and joint destruction in test animals with rheumatoid arthritis, with beneficial results[59]

~ along with other nutrients, plays a role in the prevention of prostate cancer[60,61]

~ is found in reduced quantities in those with Alzheimer's disease[62]

~ slows the decline in mental functioning that occurs with age, especially in those who consume vitamin E from food[63,64]

Gym bunnies take note: vitamin E decreases damage occurring from rigorous aerobic activity.

Minerals

I have selected only a few minerals for discussion here in the interest of brevity. It should be enough, however, to give you insight into the importance of consuming green leafy vegetables and young grass plants for their mineral values.

Potassium and Sodium

Nearly everyone who consumes the typical American diet ingests too much sodium and is deficient in potassium. The trouble is, our bodies are designed to thrive in a world where sodium is scarce and potassium abundant. And for good reason: If you look at the potassium and sodium content of most natural foods, you'll find they have plenty of potassium but little sodium. Consequently, a complex control system, good at hoarding sodium and disposing of surplus potassium, is part of our biological makeup. Study the potassium and sodium content of processed foods, and you will find the relationship between these two minerals reversed!

Why is this ratio reversal important? Back to cell membranes. While complicated proteins *control* the membrane, sodium and potassium *power* them. Each cell membrane operates a kind of electrochemical machine called the *sodium-potassium pump*.

No one knows exactly what gives the membrane the energy to pump all those ions back and forth, but we do know that by using food energy to push charged particles of potassium into the cell and sodium out, an electrical charge is maintained.

> Building this electrical potential is like charging a battery. Your cell power can now be used by thousands of different cell membrane proteins to accomplish tasks that require energy.

As often as a thousand times a second, sodium and potassium ions exchange places to inform your brain about size, distance, patterns, and color. If potassium is in short supply – or if the ratio of potassium to sodium is too low – your cell membranes become tired. Additional results of an unbalanced sodium/potassium ratio are compromised cell nourishment, reduced immune function, and lowered resistance to toxins. It can also create a feeling of puffiness and bloatedness (something we all experience when we eat too much salt.)

The solution? Make sure your diet includes lots of potassium. Most experts recommend at least three times as much potassium as sodium.[65] Some diets aimed at reducing high blood pressure suggest a ratio of 15 to 1.[66] But the typical American diet has about two to three times as much sodium as potassium — again, just the reverse of what you need!

Grain grasses typically have 100 to 200 times as much potassium as sodium, a marvelous relationship. A typical grass value is 400 to 450 milligrams of potassium per 100 grams.. This is slightly more than you find in a banana, the traditional high-potassium food. And organically grown foods tend to be much higher in potassium than non-organic foods.

You can learn more about potassium and sodium from my book, *Everything You Always Wanted to Know About Potassium But Were Too Tired to Ask.*

Calcium

Bones are not what they appear to be. That is, they are not static structures, but living tissue. A surprisingly large amount of calcium flows in and out of your bones every day. If you didn't supply your body with a constant stream of calcium, along with magnesium, phosphorus, manganese, boron, and other minerals necessary to assimilate and construct bone material, your skeleton would crumble in just a few years. This is almost exactly what happens with osteoporosis, a disease afflicting an overwhelming percentage of women in North America.

> **In the time frame during which the population of American women doubled, the incidence of osteoporosis tripled!**

But why this risky exchange of calcium in and out of bones? The answer is that your body has a very low tolerance for variations in calcium concentrations in your blood. When more calcium is needed, it has to be available *immediately* because deficiencies lead to serious problems. Complex backup systems allow calcium to be grabbed from your bones to assure the maintenance of circulating calcium in your blood. Thus your bones act as your calcium reservoir.

Doesn't milk offer an adequate supply? No, it doesn't, despite what the ads would have us believe. The calcium in commercial cow's milk almost never has a positive effect on human calcium assimilation for a number of reasons, among them:

~ an unbalanced phosphorus/calcium ratio
~ an altered fat profile
~ diminished enzymes (destroyed in the pasteurization process)

I'm sure you've heard it before, but here it is again: The fact is that cow's milk, although a superb food for calves, is a very poor food for humans. So we have yet another example of how food processing has a deleterious effect on our metabolism.

Where does all that calcium in milk come from, anyway? Do you see the farmer giving calcium pills to the cows? Mature cows never drink milk, and you won't find the farmer out in the field making them swallow calcium pills. The secret is that cows eat lots of *grass*.

Iron

> The ancient Greeks, eager to acquire strength, consumed iron shavings dissolved in vinegar. In the 15th century, iron was noted for its ability to restore "young girls when pallid, sickly and lacking color to health and beauty." (Iron nails were inserted into apples, allowed to rust, and then the apples were consumed.)[67]

Hemoglobin is a complex, giant molecule which contains, like a tiny jewel in the center of each of its four bsic components, a single atom of iron. This iron accepts the oxygen, and as it does so, develops the birght red color which differentiates oxygenated blood of the arteries from the dark red, bluish blood of the veins.

Iron has long since been associated with strength and well being (bodybuilders even "pump iron" to look like Arnold Schwarzenegger), but it is the most common mineral deficiency in the world. Iron deficiency produces a series of functional deficits beyond those ascribed to the impaired transport of oxygen to tissues.[68] Low levels of iron are associated with reduced work capacity and impaired intellectual performance. Among treatment problems is the fact that intravenous infusion of iron can precipitate joint inflammation.

Inhibitors of iron absorption are meat, whole grains, bran, and calcium phosphate. Vitamin C, however, enhances absorption.

The Zinc and Superoxide Dismutase (SOD) Connection
Many steps are involved in the process of empowering you with
energy; necessary dynamics that enable you to function – to blink,
to wave hello, to get up from a chair, to read this book, even to
smile.

A small amount of oxygen (only 1 to 2 percent) is used during
the process of energy-infusing cell metabolism, and it is left as
an *oxygen intermediate* – a substance that contributes to many
illnesses, including inflammatory diseases, toxic reactions, cancer, and aging disorders.[69]

For those who want the biochemistry, the result can be a *superoxide anion*, one of the most common oxygen intermediates.
Written as O2-, denoting two oxygen atoms with one extra elec-
tron for a negative charge, superoxide is a kind of "natural" free
radical. Superoxide and other oxygen intermediates can be used
to good advantage. Phagocytic cells, for example, use them to
surround and destroy invading cells of an infection or parasite.
(Phagocytes are blood cells that ingest foreign particles such as
bacteria.)

But every other cell in your body needs protection *against* superoxide, and the enzyme *superoxide dismutase*, as you have already learned, is the primary line of defense. SOD is an oxygen-
intermediate scavenger. Of the 100,000 enzymes in the body, SOD
ranks number five in total concentration. The theory has been
advanced by gerontologist Dr. Richard Cutter that *lifespan is directly controlled by SOD.*[70]

Zinc plays a key role in SOD metabolism. Without zinc:
~ membrane lipids would be oxidized, altering the essential internal and external cell structure
~ cellular proteins and DNA would be oxidized and damaged
~ enzymes would neutralize, shutting down cell respiration (essentially the same as killing the cell)

The big lesson we've learned in nutrition in the last few years centers on the interrelationships of nutrients. The amount of zinc in an agricultural product is closely tied to the amount found in the soil in which it was grown. Needless to say, most of the food in the supermarket vegetable section has far less of this vital mineral than the corresponding wild plant, or the plant grown under very special circumstances. Even though zinc is a trace mineral – a healthy human body has only about two grams – it's safe to say that zinc deficiency is common. Zinc is also water-soluble, so it's easily carried away by cooking water.

Zinc is needed for the synthesis of over a hundred different enzymes and has a role in male sexual functions (providing a possible explanation for the folklore associated with oysters, which are very high in zinc).

Whole grains are a good source of zinc. Note, however, that most of the zinc is in the germ and bran. Refining grain into white flour typically removes about 80 percent of this mineral.

Sources of zinc are oysters, herring, organ meats, eggs, bones, brewer's yeast, legumes, nuts, paprika, whole grains, mushrooms, and *leafy greens*.

WE KNOW THE WAY; WHERE IS THE WILL?

Our medical community is in agreement that better nutritional management of a host of chronic diseases would extend the life of the patient and reduce the chance of death from an infection.

There is also wide recognition that quality of life depends strongly on the quality of the food consumed. But I watch with horror as I observe what people put on the check-out counter at the supermarket (and even at the health food store). I have to wonder why this information is lost to the average consumer. Don't be the average consumer. Use your knowledge to maintain your health.

CHAPTER SEVEN
MORE
NUTRACEUTICALS AND
FUNCTIONAL FOODS

...in which we will learn about the amazing health benefits of a number of other substances.

We as a nation are very accustomed to relying on drugs and medicine whenever we are sick. But there is extensive evidence demonstrating that people can deal with many health problems on their own, using special products as an adjunct to their doctor's advice – products that can facilitate healing and improve immune status. We know there are several ways to cajole these healing forces into action, and we also know that they involve only that which is *natural*.

25,000 phytochemicals and more than 150,000 edible plants exist on earth. Modern humans eat only 150 to 200 of these plants worldwide, but the average American eats only 3 servings of plant foods a day, if that much.[1] The problem is that eating 5 to 9 servings of fruit and vegetables daily, as recommended by the National Cancer Institute, requires serious lifestyle changes. *But the good news is that the use of nutraceuticals does not!*

"Lifestyle" pharmacology (the prescribing of drugs to enhance life quality rather than to prevent death and disability) has become very popular for those who can afford it. Viagra, estrogen, testosterone, and human growth hormone are some examples.

But adverse drug reactions remain a leading cause of admission to hospitals and potential causes of disability and death.[2] In fact, the number of persons affected by harmful drug events in the United States is four times the total number killed in automobile accidents every year.[3] You have to wonder how this is considered progress.

Here are some examples of nutraceuticals and functional foods now popular in North America:

EFFECTIVE NUTRACEUTICALS

Food-type supplements that offer nutritional support by enhancing immunity

> barley leaf powder
> beets (crystallized)
> brewer's yeast
> colostrum
> garlic (aged)
> ginseng (Siberian)
> mushrooms (extractions)
> rice bran (stabilized)
> velvet antler

EFFECTIVE FUNCTIONAL FOODS

Foods that are health-promoting beyond their nutritional value

> eggs (fertile)
> flaxseed
> garlic
> human milk
> mushrooms (whole, not as an extract)
> Rooibos tea
> walnuts

NUTRACEUTICALS

Barley leaf powder
Because this nutraceutical is potent and easy to incorporate into your daily diet, the next chapter details one company's cutting-edge production process of young barley leaf powder, and explains its unusual additions to this product.

In addition to barley, other important cereal grasses (as greens, not as grains) include kamut and older varieties of wheat grasses. Sprouted and then dried or juiced, they are concentrated suppliers of everything that's good about vegetables. Here are descriptions of a few other significant nutraceuticals.

Beets (crystallized)
Red beet crystals are a naturally sweet tasting and instantly soluble product in an unadulterated, concentrated form. The crystals are harvested from beet tubers, mostly available from organic fields in Germany. The company producing this product is known for the purity and quality of its freshly pressed plant and vegetable juices.

> Although the beet crystals retain much of the valuable, natural elements of fresh beets, I use this product particularly to make potent nutrient mixtures more palatable.

There is something to the legend that beets are good for your blood. One of the problems with beets is that they require a lot of cooking, so most of the nutrients go down the drain. Not nearly as much is loss with these dehydrated beets.

The entire beet is used, including the fiber. Beet fiber supports healthy bacterial function in the colon, and thus can ameliorate diarrhea.[4] It can also help to eliminate abnormal cells caused by irradiation of the colon.[5]

Brewer's yeast

Yeasts are found in virtually every conceivable biological niche on the planet. Common on plant leaves and flowers, they are also found on our skin surfaces and in our intestinal tracts, where they may live symbiotically or as parasites. What are yeasts, anyway? They are single-cell living organisms, classified as fungi. Negative associations of yeast do not apply to those strains that are available naturally as food supplements.

> **Yeast cells are part of our microflora, and the right strains contribute to our health in a very positive way.**

Most of us know the strain of yeast called *Saccharomyces cerevisiae* as brewer's yeast. Saccharomyces cerevisiae has been used to prevent recurrences of *Clostridium difficile*-associated diarrhea.[6] (Clostridium difficile is a bacterium, and one of the most common causes of infection of the colon in the US, affecting millions of people annually.) Its favorable effects in supplemental form are attributed to its fermentation ability and water holding capacity in the large intestine.[7]

> **The chromium from brewer's yeast has a very beneficial effect on diabetics, more so than inorganic chromium.**

Brewer's yeast chromium offers better control of glucose, is retained more by the body, lowers triglycerides and HDL-cholesterol, and may even help some type 2 diabetics reduce and even eliminate insulin requirements.

Brewer's yeast is the richest natural so7rce containing the largest number of B vitamins.

An excellent remedy for relieving constipation is a combination of viable yogurt with brewer's yeast.[8]

Colostrum

Colostrum is the "first milk" secreted by female mammals coming into lactation. It is produced for only one to two days after giving birth, before the real milk supply starts to flow.

> ## Colostrum is loaded with immune factors, growth factors, and other specialized nutrients.

Colostrum is one of the most complex and complete nutritional substances in existence. It is also the nutritional supplement with the longest history of safe and effective use by humans. We know it is critical for the health of a newborn infant. But as a nutraceutical, it can be of benefit at any age.

The most critical components of colostrum are those that fight infection. Colostrum contains antibodies in the form of immuno-globulins, complicated molecules specially configured to bind or "stick" to specific antigens in bacteria, viruses, fungi, and certain chemical toxins, facilitating their destruction and removal by white blood cells or other components of the immune system.

Colostrum also contains:
> ~ a full complement of vitamins and minerals
> ~ *Lactobacillus bifidus*, one of the beneficial organisms that prevents the growth of other more dangerous bacteria in the intestines
> ~ chemicals that help attract the right kinds of white blood cells to sites of infection and send other chemical messages between white blood cells
> ~ important constituents of cell membranes that provide binding sites for hormones

No, we don't have to be running around pulling nursing babies off their mothers to get it. Bovine colostrum from cows (which, by the way, has immune factors almost identical to that of humans) is widely available in health food stores.

Garlic (aged)

Garlic supplements are consumed in many cultures for their cholesterol-lowering power and for their circulatory benefits. Some garlic preparations also appear to possess liver-protective, immune-enhancing, anticancer, and chemopreventive activities.

Extracts of fresh garlic – aged over a prolonged period to produce a special aged garlic extract – contain antioxidant phytochemicals known to prevent oxidant damage. It has been shown to protect against agents used in cancer therapy, against liver toxicity caused by industrial chemicals, and against the damage of acetaminophen, the popular Tylenol analgesic.

Evidence also shows that aged garlic can protect against acute damage from aging, radiation and chemical exposure.

Aged garlic reduces the risk of cardiovascular disease, stroke, and brain cell damage implicated in Alzheimer's disease.[9]

Aged garlic:
> ~ inhibits the growth of cancer cells and decreases psychological stress (determined by measuring spleen weight).[10]
> ~ may protect the small intestine from drug-induced damage.[11]
> ~ may be useful for prevention of atherosclerosis because it protects against oxidized LDL, which leads to heart disease.[12]
> ~ prevents lipid peroxide damage in a dose-dependent manner. (the more you take, the less the damage)[13]

Studies suggest that diet supplementation with aged garlic may reduce age-related learning disabilities and cognitive disorders in older people.[14] Garlic has the potential for the prevention and control of cardiovascular disease.[15]

Ginseng (Siberian)

Siberian ginseng is my favorite among ginseng varieties. Perhaps it's because I have visited the Japanese laboratories and the mountains of Hokkaido, the northernmost island of Japan, and have seen for myself that Siberian ginseng is not cultivated in an artificial environment; that it is grown and picked according to strict protocols that assure quality.

> **Compounds in Siberian ginseng show antioxidant activity, exhibit anticancer properties, and can lower cholesterol. They are also known to moderate insulin levels[16] and to reduce pain.**

As Dr. Herb Kandel points out in my book, *Hormone Replacement Therapy, Yes or No: How to Make an Informed Decision*: "Siberian ginseng is useful for increasing energy levels and promoting enhanced tolerance to stress. It is useful for menopausal women who suffer from chronic fatigue or illnesses, frequent colds or flu, and sensitivity to emotional and environmental stress. Ginseng needs to be taken on an ongoing basis for several weeks to notice the effects. Panax ginseng and Korean ginseng can elevate blood pressure and may increase endometrial build up, so these varieties should be avoided by menopausal women."[18]

Mushroom extracts

Mushrooms grow in a hostile environment. They exist at the bottom rung of the food chain, living off fallen trees and decayed material, competing with bacteria and other environmental "lowlifes."

In order for a mushroom spore to thrive, it must have an aggressive, proactive immune system, especially since mushrooms excrete their digestive enzymes *outside* of their cells. Their excretions must be able to immobilize the pathogens around them, so that the mushrooms can reabsorb the digested nutrients – uncontaminated – back into their cells.

It's no surprise, then, that fungi provide powerful immune support – especially when compared with other plant medicines.

Because more than fifty mushroom species have yielded potential immune-enhancing effects, they are being referred to as *immunoceuticals*. All are nontoxic and very well tolerated.[19]

As nutraceuticals, it is the mushroom *extracts* that we're discussing. The most super-active strains are often combined for a preventive panacea that can inject vitality into your immune system.

> When used along with chemotherapy or radiation, powerful mushroom combinations improve the effectiveness of cancer treatment, increasing remission and survival rates.

Various mushroom strains have demonstrated anticarcinogenic and antimutagenic activity,[20] antihyperglycemic and insulin-like activity,[21] the ability to help prevent cavities,[22] antioxidant components,[23] and free radical scavenging.[24] Dried shiitake mushroom powder, for example, contain high amounts of vitamin D.

You want to select natural, unprocessed, and unrefined mushroom extracts. Mushrooms can be very potent!

> Be aware that some mushroom strains may straddle a blurry boundary between nutraceutical and pharmaceutical.

It is interesting to note that mutagenic and premutagenic compounds present in mushroom are generally not heat labile (that is, not destroyed by cooking).[25]

Rice bran (stabilized)
One of the problems with cultivated cereal grains, and especially rice, is what happens to the rice after harvesting. The very basic "advantage" of agriculture is that it allows a large quantity of grain to be planted over a large area of land, and then harvested and stored. This provides a reliable and continuous food supply for the clan, tribe, village, or city.

But whole rice has a very serious shelf-life problem. *Lipase.* a natural enzyme in rice bran causes the oil to become rancid. When rice is growing, the lipase and the oil are isolated from each other, in separate types of cells. However, as soon as any mechanical processing occurs – as when rice is hulled or when the bran is removed from the kernel in the process of "polishing" white rice – the cell walls are ruptured and lipase meets rice bran oil. From there it only takes *a few hours* for the fragile components of the oil to become oxidized and rancid.

Seven thousand years ago the solution was simple: Mill the rice to remove the hull and the bran, leaving only the white kernel underneath. Now we have long shelf life, but we have also removed most of the nutrients that our bodies rely on.

Look at what's being thrown away in rice bran:

~ Gamma Oryzanol and related compounds. These are potent antioxidants and trace nutrients that play a vital role in so many aspects of human physiology that they suggest a symbiotic relationship between fresh rice and humans. *Gamma oryzanol is found only in rice bran.*

~ Tocopherals and tocotrienols, at least eight different varieties. These are all types of vitamin E, although commercial vitamin E supplements are usually in the form of alpha-tocopheral alone. The importance of the others is at least equal to that of the alpha form.

~ Polyphenols including ferulic acid, alpha-lipoic acid. Lipoic acid is believed to play an important role in sugar metabolism at the cellular level.

~ The metal chelators magnesium, calcium, and phosphorous. Also manganese and other trace minerals.

~ Phytosterols, including beta sitosterol, campesterol, stigmasterol, and at least eleven more. These are the trace nutrients that help explain why fresh vegetables are so good for you.

~ Carotenoids, including beta-carotene, alpha carotene, lycopene, lutein, zeazanthin, and more.

~ Essential amino acids including tryptophan, histidine, methionine, cystein, cystine, and argenine.

~ Nine B-vitamins, polysaccharides, and phospholipids. Phospholipids are vital to maintaining healthy cell membranes.

~ Lecithin (phosphatidyl choline and phosphatidyl serine), helpful in averting age-related mental decline.

~ Seven identified enzymes, including coenzyme Q10 and superoxidase dismutase.

The bulk, or macro-nutrients - carbohydrates, starch, sugars - are still there in white rice, of course, so the tummy feels full. But white rice is a nutritional wasteland.

What about brown rice? Brown rice is brown because a layer of rice bran is left in place. But the hulling process still causes enough disruption to release lipase into the bran. The result is that virtually all brown rice contains rancid oils to some degree. The long-held belief that brown rice is nutritionally superior to white rice is suddenly called into question.

Rice bran has been used as a nutraceutical for as long as rice has been grown. Even in modern India, it is not uncommon for the mother of a sick child to collect some fresh bran from rice polishings to use as a therapeutic tea for a sick child. But the bran has to be very fresh, or it is worthless. Because it has been so hard to stabilize this nutrient-rich food, millions of tons of it are discarded or sold for low-grade animal feed every year.

This situation has dramatically changed, and supplements derived from stabilized rice bran are showing enormous therapeutic value. New processes have been developed that reliably denature the lipase in rice bran without causing very much damage to the rest of the rice bran's chemistry. The result is a stabilized rice bran product that retains most of the vital nutrients of fresh rice bran, but has a shelf life measured in years rather than hours.

Stabilized rice bran is available in several forms, with various ratios of soluble to insolube components and other nutraceutical additives. They all share the surprisingly pleasant nutty taste of fresh rice bran, and the safety of a food that's been used by humans for thousands of years.

Although this is a new entrant in the nutraceutical field, stabilized rice bran is rapidly accumulating an impressive body of positive results from laboratory research and clinical trials

Some of the most promising uses are against diabetes, arthritis, peripheral neuropathy, high cholesterol and cardiovascular disease. While the exact modes of action are often unclear, many of these chronic conditions have their indirect origins in oxidative damage. It is likely that the right antioxidant at the right time is what is really responsible for the broad-spectrum efficacy of stabilized rice bran.

Stabilized rice bran is one of the nutraceuticals that will help reverse our civilization's 10,000 year decline in nutritional quality.

Velvet antler

Deer antler sounds like the kind of ingredient that should go into the cauldron along with "eye of newt" and "toe of frog." At first impression, the uninformed might be tempted to put the users of antler products far out on the nutritional lunatic fringe. And yet this substance has a credible history of effective use in Chinese herbal medicine that goes back at least two millennia. It continues to be widely used in China, Korea, Japan, and Russia.

Antlers are nothing like rhinoceros horns or tiger's teeth. Elk and deer antlers regenerate every year, and are probably the fastest growing animal tissue known. In fact, antler is the only mammalian bone structure that regenerates annually. "Velvet" antler, the form used for nutritional purposes, is harvested from the deer or elk without doing any harm to the animal. Unlike the inert and calcified horn or tooth; velvet antler is loaded with growth and immune factors, cartilage, glucosamine sulfate, chondroitin sulfate, and collagen.

The last three substances are currently in favor by those seeking a natural remedy for arthritis. Even the FDA recognizes the effectiveness of chondroitin and collagen, allowing structure and function claims for joint health. But when these substances are naturally packaged in velvet antler, the various co-factors seem to result in a significant performance edge over the isolated chemicals when it comes to repairing damaged joints.

Velvet antler can sometimes have a pronounced positive effect on male sexuality. While anecdotal reports are common, controlled trials have been sparse and controversial. But it is not unusual for science to lag behind practice, and we are close enough to the anecdotes to see why velvet antler can, under some circumstances, legitimately be referred to as "natural Viagra." This aspect of velvet antler has probably hindered more than helped the recognition of antler's value, because aphrodisiacs tend to be stigmatized, or at best not taken seriously.

Velvet antler is also one of a very few natural sources for IGF-I and II, the secondary hormones that do the work for human growth hormone. These are probably the substances responsible for increased effectiveness of chondroitin sulfate and glucosamine sulfate in velvet antler.

For millions of years, humans and human ancestors ate nearly all of the animals they killed. Blood, brains, organ meat, connective tissue, bone marrow, and every body part were all consumed, and consumed raw. And it's interesting to note that wild predators rarely leave much behind when they make a kill – bones included

It is only in the last century or two that non-meat animal components have been left off the plate. Velvet antler is a practical way of putting back some of the things that we're missing, things that our bodies are designed to thrive on. We can't bring whole fresh-killed animals home to our kitchens, even if we wanted to. But we can take antler supplements.

Is it possible that many of our chronic health problems are related to throwing away the most valuable parts of our food?

As explained in my book, *The Remarkable Healing Power of Velvet Antler,* this substance is being used today for arthritis relief, muscle development, increased strength, increased endurance, red blood cell production to correct anemia, capacity of blood to carry oxygen, speedy recovery from injury and stress, faster recuperation after surgery, augmented levels of certain anabolic hormones, enhanced immune activity, and fertility.[26]

Perhaps the potion boiling in the caldron with the "eye of newt" and "toe of frog" would be a better brew than we imagine.

FUNCTIONAL FOODS

Eggs
The myth that avoiding eggs helps to reduce the risk of heart disease is just that – a myth! An egg is an excellent example of a functional food.

Eggs are a fantastic dietary source of many essential components that promote optimum health. Among the nutrients found in eggs: quality protein, choline (which promotes memory and brain function), plus lutein and zeaxanthin (nutrients that help prevent cataracts). Egg yolks can be a source of docosahexaenoic acid (DHA – a beneficial fatty acid found mostly in fish oils), plus vitamin D and iron – not found in too many other foods.[27]

It is gratifying to researchers like myself to see scientific validation from the traditional medical community for concepts we have had for decades. Eggs make an important contribution to the diet. And they are relatively inexpensive and versatile!

> There's no question that the egg will continue to play an important role in the changing face of functional foods.[28]

Flaxseed
Once upon a time, every town and hamlet had its own oil mill. Many plants and seeds were used, but the favorite for producing oil was flaxseed. It had a nutty, rich, almost creamy flavor, which tasted a lot like fresh butter.

As hamlets grew to towns and towns to cities, it became commonplace to have fresh oil delivered door-to-door, just as milk, eggs, and butter were in later days, or water today. Flaxseed oil was sold in small quantities and used only if fresh. People understood just how its health-sustaining and therapeutic values worked best.

But oil-making practices changed with the use of machinery and specialization – efforts that made daily chores less arduous. Small presses were replaced with automated, continuous-feed inventions. These were run at rates and pressures that raised the temperature of the oil far above the boiling point. Hydrocarbon solvents extracted more flaxseed oil at a faster rate. The oil was also bleached, degummed, and deodorized to extend shelf life. Heat, light, air, and time provoked rancidity. So flaxseed oil, because it was no longer a "pure" and health-promoting product, eventually disappeared from the marketplace, taken over by corn and soy oil, among others.

> As we gained knowledge, we became aware that fresh flaxseed oil contained two fatty acids not manufactured in the human body: *linoleic acid* (LA) and *linolenic acid* (LNA). The only way to get these fatty acids is to eat them. That's why they are called *essential*.

We also learned that LA and LNA are precursors – chemical building blocks of a large class of more elaborate fatty acids. These, in turn, are building blocks of literally thousands of enzymes, hormones, and prostaglandins – with many cellular functions, including bone formation. *Arachidonic acid*, made from LA, regulates viral infection and promotes resistance to toxins. Derivatives of LNA reduce the risk of fatal heart attacks and help to manufacture substances that control and limit blood platelet aggregation (the "sticking together" of blood platelets).

High in magnesium (necessary for vitamin D conversion), flax is also rich in lecithin, unmatched as a natural source of omega-3 fatty acids, and has the components needed for effective prostaglandin function. Flaxseed also produces high concentrations of lignans, known to be protective against breast cancer and to improve the ratios of progesterone and estradiol during menstruation.

The good news is that flaxseed is back in town! Organic, unadulterated, non-rancid flaxseed is available. Add to salads, soups, or nutrient "cocktail" drinks. It must be ground, however, so use a small coffee grinder and grind the whole seeds for about eight seconds, as needed. Beware of store-bought ground seeds, or oil preparations. Flax seed rancidifies quickly once ground.

Garlic

As a functional food, the information that follows pertains to a clove of garlic, as used in the kitchen for food preparation (rather than encapsulated or in tableted forms). Although garlic has been used for its medicinal properties for thousands of years, investigations into its mode of action are relatively recent.

> Garlic has a wide spectrum of actions; not only is it antibacterial, antiviral, antifungal and antiprotozoal, but it also has beneficial effects on your cardiovascular and immune systems.[29]

As explained in my book on female sexuality, *She's Gotta Have It,* both the ancient Jews and Romans worshiped the aphrodisiac powers of garlic. It was put in the same category as wine. Because it appeared to protect against infection and disease, it was interpreted as a magical substance. (Thus the legendary link to protection from evil creatures such as vampires.) Unlike other aphrodisiacs, which are known to have temporary and immediate arousal effects, garlic is said to create a long-lasting result.

In a small European town, a study was done to determine whether those with normal blood pressure consume more garlic in their diets. The average garlic eaten in this particular group turned out to be 134 grams per person monthly. Sixty-seven percent used garlic in cooked food, while the rest ate it raw or pickled. Those with blood pressure on the lower side were found to consume more garlic. (The results were statistically significant for systolic blood pressure only.)[30]

More good news:

~ Chronic garlic intake augments your own body's antioxidants, which might have important direct effects on your heart.[31]

~ A host of studies provides compelling evidence that garlic is an effective inhibitor of cancer. Studies reveal that the benefits of garlic are not limited to a specific species, to a particular tissue, or to a specific carcinogen. As is the case with nutraceuticals and functional foods in general, more than one compound is responsible for the anticancer properties associated with garlic.[32]

Human milk

This is undoubtedly the quintessential functional food, and lucky for the babies who are breast fed for at least a year or more.. "Breast is best," is what every pregnant woman now hears . . . finally! (In my day, the doctors told us that our babies would be better off with formula.)

Human milk protects against childhood obesity,[33] has beneficial effects on children's cognitive development,[34] may reduce the risk of asthma,[35] may protect children from leukemia,[36] improves the health of low-birth weight babies,[37] cuts the risk of developing lower respiratory tract infections,[38] lowers incidence, prevalence, and duration of individual episodes of diarrhea,[39] protects against celiac disease (sensitivity to gluten-containing foods, the protein found in wheat),[40] and places children at a lower risk for sudden infant death syndrome (SIDS).[41]

An interesting law prohibits the use of federal funds to "...implement, administer, or enforce any prohibition on women breast-feeding their children in Federal buildings or on Federal property."

The process of breast-feeding will lower Mom's blood pressure (if it's too high) and reduce her risk of developing breast cancer.[42]

Mushrooms

Many of the benefits of mushroom extracts apply to the whole mushroom itself. For example, the white button mushroom can inhibit an enzyme that plays a negative role in breast cancer development.

Just be sure the mushrooms you buy are organic. If they aren't, they are likely to be very heavily sprayed. Pesticides actually interfere with the inhibition of the enzyme that promotes breast cancer.

Rooibos tea

People who drink tea have better health than those who don't, and those who drink Rooibos tea fare even better.

The constituents in Rooibos have been scientifically documented to relieve insomnia, nervous tension, depression, stomach cramps (including colic), constipation, and allergy symptoms (even those caused by hay fever and asthma). It can also ease itching and skin irritations, thereby offering eczema and acne victims welcome deliverance from misery. *And all this is the least of its health-giving capacities!*

Iron is reduced by about one-third in tea drinkers.[43] The culprit? Tannin. Tannins (commonly referred to as tannic acid) can also decrease growth rate and protein digestibility. Foods rich in tannins are considered to be of low nutritional value.[44] A study was carried out to determine if Rooibos tea has a deleterious effect on iron absorption similar to that of ordinary tea. The conclusion: Rooibos tea had no significant effect on iron absorption.[45]

> The low levels of tannin in Rooibos tea also make it sweeter than regular tea, for it's the tannins that make tea taste somewhat bitter.

Unlike other uplifting or "entertainment" beverages, Rooibos tea has no caffeine. Caffeine in your morning coffee puts your body in a state of sustained stress, affecting both blood pressure and heart rate all through the day. Cutting back on caffeine may be a way to reduce hypertension and heart disease.[46]

The Rooibos leaves are grown high in the mountains of South Africa, one of the few places left in the world boasting unpolluted air and unpolluted soil. Like other plants growing this way, they are extravagantly rich in naturally occurring nutrients. At a particular point in the plant's ripening process, the leaves develop a reddish brown color, which explains why this increasingly popular beverage is also referred to as "redbush" tea.

Several studies show that rooibos tea contains innumerable highly defensive natural antioxidants.[47,48] Equally exciting, Rooibos tea has been validated to have anti-aging properties. When the protective effects of Rooibos tea against damage to the central nervous system accompanying aging were examined, results suggested that ongoing intake of this elixir prevents age-related accumulation of lipid peroxides in several regions of the brain.[49]

The tea was also able to inhibit the cancer-causing effect of X-rays in test animals.

Carcinogenic transformation of cells was reduced with increased concentration of Rooibos extract. (Green tea, although also a highly rated functional food, does not have this capacity.)[50]

Walnuts
There is now scientific evidence showing a beneficial relationship between the consumption of walnuts and the reduction and prevention of coronary heart disease. Compared to most other nuts, which contain monounsaturated fatty acids, walnuts are unique because they are rich in omega-6 (linoleate) and omega-3 (linolenate) polyunsaturated fatty acids.

Walnuts contain numerous healthful components, such as having a low lysine/arginine ratio and high levels of arginine, folate, fiber, and polyphenols.

Though walnuts are energy rich, they do not cause weight gain, even when eaten as a replacement food.

Studies demonstrating these results show that daily consumption of small amounts of nuts, including walnuts, reduce your risk of coronary heart disease. It is best to purchase organic nuts in the shell, and crack as needed. Or buy shelled nuts provided they are organic and untreated, and from a source that has a quick turnover.

~ ~ ~

Think about combining functional foods, whenever possible. Here's an easy (and healthful!) lunch idea: organic mixed greens, a handful of organic walnut pieces, a light dusting of garlic grape seed oil, and a tablespoon of freshly ground flaxseed. Delicious! Just be sure the walnuts are *organic* and *fresh*.[51]

Many additional functional foods could be added to this list, including *prebiotics* (non-digestible food ingredients that stimulate bacteria in the colon) and *probiotics* (foods that contain "friendly" live bacteria). Prebiotics and probiotics comprise a powerful strategy designed to improve human health by conferring beneficial effects through your gastrointestinal tract.[52]

The main prebiotic agents consist of oligosaccharides and dietary fibers. Prebiotics escape enzymatic digestion in the upper gastrointestinal tract.[53]

More about prebiotics and probiotics in the next chapter.

Drugs deplete nutrients and undermine health:

~ Estrogen lowers zinc
~ Aspirin lowers vitamin C
~ Antacids lower all Bs
~ Diuretics lower folic acid
~ Antibiotics interfere with A and K
~ Laxatives affect A, D, and K
~ Antidepressants affect B6
~ Gout drugs affect vitamin B
~ Corticosteroids reduce vitamin C
~ Hypotensives decrease B6
~ Oral contraceptives decrease B vitamins
~ Tamoxifen increases endometrial cancer
~ Antacids and acid-lowering drugs increase absorption of toxins
~ Anti-inflammatory drugs interfere with the liver's ability to get rid of toxins

Alcohol depletes nutrients. Every drink you take causes: thiamine loss, impaired vitamin B6 activation, folate loss, and increased magnesium excretion.

The octogenarian of today is too often frail, immobile, incontinent, and intellectually impaired. Unfortunately, seniors represent the fastest growing population in developed countries at this time.

Perhaps this is one reason that aging jokes proliferate. But humor is not always an exaggeration of reality. An example:

Why is celebrating your first and last birthday so similar?

Answer:
~ You can't eat all the foods served.
~ Someone has to feed you.
~ You don't recognize all the people present.
~ You need help blowing out the candles.

As we begin to slowly unravel the conundrums of cellular communication, nutrient re-uptake, feedback mechanisms, information molecules, peptide actions, neurochemical metabolism – to say nothing of the interconnections of all of these goings-on – we keep getting closer to what we need to know in our search for immune competence and wellness as we age.

But it appears that the bottom line will always be the same. The simple answer is:
   nutraceuticals and functional foods.

CHAPTER EIGHT
WE *CAN*
CONCENTRATE NATURE

...in which we explain probiotics and prebiotics – as well as discuss the importance of lactic acid bacteria, oligosaccharides, and fiber, and how they enhance an already great powdered barley leaf nutraceutical.

This book has shown you exactly how the barley leaf provides so many of the nutritional advantages that make nutraceuticals and functional foods special. And as close to perfect as the barley leaf is, one company has gone a step further: it has taken the barley leaf and added a few select nutraceuticals – lactic acid bacteria (or lactobacillus, known as acidophilus), soluble fiber, and oligosaccharides – to the mix. We will discuss this amazing product at the end of this chapter.

PROBIOTICS – THE ARMY WITHIN

Antibiotic has been a household word for decades. We all know it has something to do with killing or inhibiting the growth of undesirable microorganisms, the kind you *don't* want in your body. *Probiotic*, on the other hand, means "promoting life," and has only recently become part of our medical vocabulary.

Probiotics refer to food supplements that *promote* the growth and proliferation of the kind of microorganisms you *do* want inside your body, the bacteria that are vital to your health and wellness. They have been defined as viable (live) microorganisms that, when ingested, have a beneficial effect in the prevention and treatment of specific pathologic conditions.

> Probiotics exert their effects through a phenomenon known as *colonization resistance,* whereby huge numbers of the friendly flora in your digestive tract limit the concentration of potentially pathogenic flora.[1]

As an average adult, you have about 100 trillion bacteria living in your intestinal tract – *adding up to about four pounds of living material!* Approximately 400 different species are represented. This complex mass of life forms – an entire ecosystem in miniature – is so vital to your health that it's often thought of as an organ in its own right.

At home primarily in your intestinal tract, these microorganisms help with digestion and elimination, as well as contribute certain vitamins, enzymes, and specialized "natural" antibiotics. Probiotics are also responsible for some very specific functions in disease resistance.

Here are some of the most important roles probiotics play in the body:

Production of important digestive enzymes
Probiotics counteract lactose intolerance by their association with lactase, which breaks down otherwise indigestible milk sugars. This digestive enzyme helps to replace the natural food enzymes destroyed during cooking.[2]

Intercepting carcinogenic substances before they are absorbed
Probiotics cause toxins to be destroyed or eliminated instead of assimilated.

Some probiotics may even produce enzymes that degrade nitro-samines, a carcinogenic substance found in many processed foods and beverages (especially rampant in processed meats like hot dogs and bologna).

Detoxification
By binding to unwanted metabolites and causing them to be ex-creted, probiotics help with detoxification.

Immune protection
Probiotics support immune functions of the intestinal tract lining by protecting the surfaces of mucous membranes. They help to suppress undesirable bacteria by maintaining an antibacterial and antifungal environment.[3]

Reduction of bad breath
Probiotics replace organisms responsible for unpleasant mouth odors, and also reduce flatulence by breaking down the sugars that promote methane-producing bacteria.[4] (So you can thank probiotics for your next date!)

Cholesterol control
By promoting normal absorption of dietary fats and facilitating elimination of unwanted cholesterol before it is absorbed, probiotics help to keep cholesterol at normal, safe levels.[5]

Production of nutrients
Probiotics promote the production of additional supplies of vita-mins and other trace nutrients. Many of the B vitamins (includ-ing riboflavin, B12, thiamine, folic acid, and pantothenic acid), in addition to certain proteins, are produced by probiotics.[6]

Suppression of certain infections
Probiotics claim suppression of Candida, urinary tract infections, and a number of other intestinal disorders.[7]

Diarrhea control in infants and children
There is evidence of significant benefit of probiotics in the treatment of acute infectious diarrhea in infants and children.[8] The favorable clinical effect of lactic acid, especially in children, has now been positively demonstrated.[9]

The health benefits of probiotics have been recognized for thousands of years by people the world over, and have withstood the test of time.[10]

Traditional societies continue to include cultured food products as an important part of their diet. But today, the commercial versions of most of these foods are almost completely lacking in viable organisms, and probiotics are just about nonexistent in the American diet. In the forms available to us, the bacteria that cause the fermentation of the food – the ones we want in our intestinal tract – are barely capable of multiplying into the billions of living microorganism we need. Even commercial yogurt rarely contains effective live cultures.

My grandmother "clabbered" milk and drank kefir. Do you have any idea what your ancestors may have done as part of the health wisdom they inherited through the ages? Bulgarians eat yogurt; Germans, sauerkraut; Asians, tempeh, miso, tamari, pickled daikon, or kimchee; Africans ferment millet; various cultures ferment both vegetables and grains.

In our culture today, in addition to lacking an effective source food for appropriate intestinal organisms, it is also more difficult to *maintain* intestinal flora even after it has been established. This may be a result of poor diet, but preservatives, additives, and pesticide residues are also directly responsible. Antibiotic drugs or treatments are particularly damaging to intestinal bacteria, and the effects can last for weeks after their use is discontinued.

With such a vast army of life forms ready to do so much to protect us, it's amazing that most Americans fail to make use of this important health strategy. But those "in the know" turn to probiotic supplements or foods. Probiotics work best when taken on a regular basis. A bowl of viable cultured yogurt (usually meaning home-made) is one great source.

If you are lactose intolerant, you may already have demonstrated the effectiveness of a probiotic by your tolerance to viable yogurt compared with milk.[11]

You could also have a serving of sauerkraut (minus the preservatives, not easy to find), which will send billions of bacteria into your digestive system, like tiny soldiers ready to fight for your good health. An easier solution? At least one brand of young barley leaf powder that has *lactic acid bacteria* added to it!

> Since harmful bacteria colonize almost out of control in hospital settings, it's a good idea to be well fortified with probiotics before any hospital visit.

Lactic Acid Bacteria, a Probiotic

Lactic acid bacteria (lactobacilli) are widely used in yogurt and other dairy products.

These organisms are nonpathogenic and nontoxic, and they retain their viability during storage. They also survive passage through the stomach and small bowel.

Lactic acid bacteria have been present in food since the early days of civilization. Byproducts of these bacteria inhibit the growth of several important pathogens and increase shelf life beyond current "chemical" preservatives.

Because lactic acid bacteria already preserve foods such as cheese and milk, the food chemists believe it makes sense to try and inoculate them into other foods as well. Besides being less potentially toxic or carcinogenic than current antimicrobial agents, lactic acid bacteria are more effective and flexible in several applications. According to *Current Opinions in Microbiology*, detailed knowledge of their physiological traits may lead to potential new applications for these organisms in the food industry (especially for preservation), while other traits are beneficial for human health.[12]

On a personal level, lactic acid bacteria keep your pH ratio (acid-alkaline balance) at its optimum level. A low pH (less than 4.5) can prevent the growth of unwanted bacteria. Lactic acid bacteria should predominate in certain body fluids to help the fermentation of the "good-guy" bacteria – the bacteria that fight germs. For example, a decrease of lactic acid bacteria in vaginal fluid can lead to vaginitis (an inflammation of the vaginal mucosa, resulting from infection).[13]

Medical definition of lactic acid bacteria: *a group of bacteria that carry out a lactic acid fermentation of sugars. It includes species of* Lactobacillus, Leuconostoc, Pediococcus *and* Streptococcus.

Lactic acid bacteria are among the best-studied microorganisms. Here are just a few reports I found compelling:

~ Lactic acid bacteria eaten at breakfast has the potential to improve glucose tolerance of food eaten four hours later, even if the lunch is a high-glycemic meal.[14] A high glycemic meal is one that is high in carbohydrates – the kind that will normally adversely affect your blood sugar level. (In addition to diabetics, athletes and those who are overweight can benefit from understanding the concept involved.)

~ Lactic acid bacteria inhibit unfavorable bacterial strains.[15]

~ Lactic acid bacteria are effective in reducing *E. coli* and other harmful bacteria, so it could be useful as a pathogen intervention step in meat production. It has the potential to keep meat free of infectious diseases.[16]

> We are becoming increasingly aware that properly formulated, probiotic-containing foods offer a dietary component with the potential to promote health in a variety of ways.[17]

PREBIOTICS

Prebiotics are non-digestible food ingredients that can stimulate the growth or activities of probiotic-like bacteria normally present in the colon, thereby improving health. To be effective, prebiotics should escape digestion in the upper gut, reach the large bowel, and be utilized selectively. The food ingredients most likely to meet these criteria are oligosaccharides (but not all oligosaccharides have prebiotic properties).

Among these properties, prebiotics can:
          ~ provide a healthy colonic environment
          ~ enhance resistance to invading pathogens
          ~ provide non-specific stimulation of immune function
          ~ reduce the production of LDL production
          ~ increase absorption of calcium and magnesium

> Prebiotics are also antimutagenic. And because they are not glycemic (that is, they don't raise blood sugar), they are potentially useful for diabetics.

Oligosaccharides, a Prebiotic

Many years ago, on a visit to Asia, I discovered that oligosaccharides were widely used in Japanese food products. Because of the superior health of the Japanese, I investigated further, and wrote the first article for American consumers explaining the benefits of this food ingredient. Not surprisingly, it took us *years* to catch up to the wisdom of incorporating oligosaccharides into our food . . . and we still have a long way to go!

I learned that fermentation of oligosaccharides in the colon results in a large number of effects, including: an increase in calcium absorption, an increased fecal weight, a potential lowering of blood lipid levels, and a shortening of gastrointestinal transit time. Transit time refers to the time it takes for food to enter your mouth, go through the digestive system, and then be eliminated, Transit time for a healthy person should be two to three days. The transit time of the average senior in this country is *two weeks.*

Oligosaccharides are found naturally – although in small quantities – in foods such as wheat, onions, bananas, honey, garlic, leeks, and artichokes.

Other effects include an increase in bifidobacteria in the colon, which is believed to benefit human health by producing compounds that inhibit potential pathogens. It does this by reducing blood ammonia levels along with producing vitamins and digestive enzymes.[18] Oligosaccharides actually stimulate the growth of these beneficial bifidobacteria, suggesting potential colon tumor inhibitory properties.[19]

Although the oligosaccharide is non-digestible, it is fermented by some of your intestinal microflora. That's how it stimulates the growth and activity of bacteria with favorable consequences.

Oligosaccharides stimulate absorption of several minerals and improve mineralization of bone. Studies with test animals show that they increase the availability of magnesium, zinc, and iron (in addition to calcium). The effects appear to depend on the ingested dose.[20] And this prebiotic also lowers pH.[21]

> Since this prebiotic helps nonviable food components to be specifically fermented in the colon by bacteria believed to be of positive value, you can see why it increases the value of young green barley powder.[22]

FIBER

The fact that we get so little fiber in the American diet is something *everyone* should be aware of. Fiber was not appreciated until recent years, mainly because it is the part of food that was assumed to play no role in our health. It is not digested, passes through the large intestine virtually unchanged, does not provide energy or nutrients or materials for growth and repair, and contains almost no calories.

As I explain in the book I wrote about fiber more than ten years ago (*New Facts About Fiber: How Fiber Supplements Can Enhance Your Health*), you can profit from knowing about the incredible correlation between health and fiber. Among the causes of a long list of diseases, there is almost always *a lack of fiber.*

Denis Burkitt, a British surgeon studying the diets of rural Africans, inspired me to write that book when I interviewed him twenty years ago on my New York City radio show. He made an amazing discovery after comparing the size of hospitals with the size of excreted feces. His finding?

> Large stools, small hospitals;
> small stools, large hospitals.

A good diet, with a high fiber content, creates bigger, more bulky stools. Processed and fast foods create what Hippocrates, more than two thousand years ago, termed "button stools."

Fiber is generally divided into two types — insoluble and soluble. Although most foods contain both types of fiber, one or the other usually predominates.

Examples of insoluble fibers (which do not dissolve in water) are hemicellulose, cellulose, and lignin, found in whole grains and certain vegetables such as barley leaf. Soluble fibers (which do dissolve in water) are found in oat bran, apples, beans, and psyllium seed husks (used as a laxative).

Unfortunately, America's eating habits have not altered significantly in any meaningful way, in spite of our increasing knowledge of the importance of fiber. Sadly, many important health messages get lost on their way to the table.

Check your fiber knowledge:

Which one of each of these foods has more fiber?

1. celery or broccoli?
2. apples or pears?
3. prunes, dates, or figs?
4. white rice or brown rice?
5. 1/2 cup of beans or 1/2 cup of peas?
6. chicken or beef?
7. yogurt or milk?

(No cheating. The answers are on the next page.)

Answers to Fiber Quiz::

1. broccoli, even though celery is crispier
2. pears
3. figs, which are especially high in fiber
4. brown rice (of course)
5. beans
6. trick question: neither — there is no fiber in any animal product
7. trick question: neither — there is no fiber in any animal product

My attention to fiber took a quantum leap after my first clinical experience. As a newly appointed nutrition consultant in a doctor's office, I recommended a daily bowl of whole-grain cereal to a patient who, at the age of thirty-one, had been on medication for constipation relief more than half her life. Three weeks later, she returned to my office, smiling broadly. "It was so simple," she said. "Just a bowl of cereal. Why didn't anyone ever tell me about cereal fiber before?"

Medical studies now offer clear and compelling evidence explaining the consequences of too little fiber, as well as the benefits of healthy levels of fiber. The crucial importance of fiber is a confirmed scientific and medical fact.

Soluble Fiber
~ lowers cholesterol
~ reduces heart disease risk
~ controls blood sugar
~ lowers blood pressure
~ promotes growth of
   friendly flora

Insoluble Fiber
~ aids digestion
~ aids elimination
~ promotes regularity
~ contributes to
   bowel cleansing

Fiber, like lactic acid bacteria and oligosaccharides, also helps the growth of healthful flora in your intestines. A few interesting facts about fiber:

~ Dietary fiber is particularly low in away-from-home eating patterns among well-educated, higher-income women.[23]
~ Calcium supplementation inhibits magnesium absorption on a fiber-free diet, but has little effect on magnesium absorption when fiber is present. Absorption of calcium is increased by including some fiber in the diet.[24]
~ A diet containing fiber encourages the excretion of food carcinogens.[25]
~ Fiber helps prevent the growth of disease-causing bacteria.
~ Fiber-rich foods protect against breast cancer.
~ Dietary fiber is considered a functional food when it imparts a special function to that food aside from the normal expected function, and when it is used as an additive. So it's a funcitonal food when it contributes to lactobacillus stimulation in the gut.
~ The reduction in serum lipid risk factors for heart disease supports the FDAs approval of a health claim for dietary fiber.
~ Fiber has the potential to prevent colorectal cancer.
~ Straining to pass small firm stools is a major cause of varicose veins (caused by fiber deficiency in the diet).
~ The greater your fiber consumption, the higher your caloric waste.

ORGANICALLY GROWN, ORGANICALLY GREEN

I have discussed the relationship of the nutrients in the young barley leaf and how they enhance your immune system. I have also explained the benefits of nutraceuticals and functional foods, why they are far superior to isolated nutrients, and why the young green barley leaf can be used as a model for *all* nutraceuticals

The fact that barley has been under-used in this country is an advantage: *it is not a product that will incite allergy.*

The exceptional attributes of the nutrient content of the young barley leaf have been defined both in general and specifically, including the high content of superoxide dismutase, chlorophyll, carotenes, enzymes, polyphenols, friendly bacteria, as well as the crucial antioxidants.

A few interesting barley green facts

~ Barley grass is slightly easier to digest than wheat grass. People allergic to wheat almost always tolerate barley grass.[26]

~ Spinach has an alkalinity of 39.6. Barley green is as high as 66.4.

~ Barley green is one of the highest natural sources of the very important enzyme superoxide dismutase (SOD).

~ If you can't get your children (or even yourself!) to eat enough green leafy vegetables, barley greens are the answer.

~ Kale, a competing green product, does not taste nearly as good as barley.

~ Some barley products may be juiced first, and then freeze-dried. Juice is good, but why throw away the non-liquid portions of the plant? I prefer to use the whole food, so I favor products based on the whole leaf.

All of this information points to two very important questions:

What kind of barley leaf supplement should I use and where can I get it?

Personally, I have been impressed with one company's product, imported from Japan. The American version is called *Shizen Green* and the Japanese original variety is known as *Ryokko Aojiru*. (The American version is slightly sweeter to accommodate the American palate.)

Both varieties include a combination of oligosaccharides, lactic acid bacteria, and fiber. The American version has green tea added as well, and both varieties are now available in the US. Many of the studies cited in this book are based on research using Shizen Green and/or Ryokko Aojiru.

Shizen green and Ryokko Aojiru are among the most meticulously produced products I have ever encountered. A windbreak forest surrounds and protects this company's crop from any agricultural chemicals. The initial planting is in a secluded and unpolluted area, and the laboratory and production facilities are precise and pristine.

The lactobacillus bacteria are grown carefully in a highly sterile environment. After the barley is processed, natural fiber (not genetically modified) is added. Since the barley leaf contains mostly insoluble fiber, the company has added soluble fiber to the mix. Even the packaging is extremely convenient and designed to effectively retain nutrient content.

You can learn more about these products by going to their website at
www.shizengreen.com
or by calling 1-866-438-4733.

CHAPTER NINE
GRAINS AS VEGETABLES OR GRAINS AS DRUGS?

...in which we reveal some uncomfortable facts about comfort foods.

Bread – the staff of life. The foundation of food pyramids, the most basic staple, and the epitome of wholesome food. But is it really? Why, when, and where did bread-making become such an important part of western culture, and is it really what our bodies are best adapted to consume? Is it even good for us at all?

Consider two important elements of baking: time and temperature. Start with any nutrient-rich food, whether leaf or seed, then bake in a preheated 450° oven for an hour. Do you think there will be any vitamins, enzymes, or tocotrienols left intact? Of course not.

Does bread-making save labor?

Consider the process from a human resources point of view: Harvesting, threshing, milling, mixing, finding fuel for the oven. Compare this to picking and eating a wild plant. Agriculture is a lot of work, and there is now consensus among anthropologists that ancient populations took up agriculture not by choice but by necessity, and that they even reverted back to hunting and gathering if they had the opportunity. Our farmer of 10,000 years ago was right!

The evidence for this is fairly clear: Nearly all hunter-gatherer societies have a good working understanding of agriculture. Some Native Americans, for example, cultivated tobacco but not food. Other ancient cultures made only temporary transitions to farming, but reverted to hunting and gathering when their situations improved.

An interview on "The Paleolithic Diet and Its Modern Implications," brought an interesting response from Loren Cordain, PhD, a professor at the Department of Exercise & Sports Science, Colorado State University, Fort Collins, Colorado. Dr Cordain said:

> The fossil record indicates that early farmers, compared to their hunter-gatherer predecessors, had a characteristic reduction in stature, an increase in infant mortality, a reduction in life span, an increased incidence of infectious diseases, an increase in iron deficiency anemia, an increased incidence of osteomalacia, porotic hyperostosis and other bone mineral disorders and an increase in the number of dental caries and enamel defects. Early agriculture did not bring about increases in health, but rather the opposite.
>
> A number of environmental pressures may have forced humans to adopt agriculture, including increases in human population densities and the depletion of easily hunted game. The extinction of large mammals all over Northern Europe, Asia, and North America coincide with the adoption of agriculture.[1]

There are many competing theories that attempt to explain the permanent transition to agriculture and the cultural "advances" that come with it. But one of the most intriguing theories is as simple as it is unexpected: bread – and in fact most products made from cereal grains – are addictive.

A paper titled "The Origins of Agriculture," by Greg Wadley and Angus Martin, in Melbourne Australia, makes the case:

> The modern human diet is very different from that of closely related primates and, almost certainly, early hominids. Though there is controversy over what humans ate before the development of agriculture, the diet certainly did not include cereals and milk in appreciable quantities.
>
> Groups led by Zioudrou and Brantl found opioid activity in wheat, maize and barley (exorphins), and bovine and human milk (casomorphin), as well as stimulatory activity in these proteins, and in oats, rye and soy. Cereal exorphin is much stronger than bovine casomorphin, which in turn is stronger than human casomorphin.
>
> Mycroft et al. estimated that 150 milligrams of the MIF-1 analogue could be produced by normal daily intake of cereals and milk, noting that such quantities are orally active, and half this amount "has induced mood alterations in clinically depressed subjects."
>
> Hence we may ask, do these findings mean that cereals and milk are chemically rewarding? Are humans somehow "addicted" to these foods?[2]

The question is answered by the data presented in the paper. Yes, there is a high enough concentration of exorphins in cereal grass grains to be psychoactive when eaten in normal quantities. This gives a whole new meaning to "comfort foods" based on pastas and breads, and might go a long way to explain why so much of the world lives on grain when intensive vegetable gardening of the same land could produce more and better food with less work.

Fear and Loathing in the Supermarket

Now that we feel less comfortable about certain comfort foods, the problem is one of adapting our daily food environment without having to summon up supernatural levels of self-discipline. If you are like me, you will not give up bread and pasta without a fight.

Fear — fear of pain, disease, and death — are powerful motivators. But they only work for the short term, when the pain is present or the disease is imminent.

Take away the pain or the frightening diagnosis, and the motivation to maintain a healthy lifestyle goes away too.

For the long run, it is the great feeling of health, energy, and vitality that will keep you true to what you already know about good nutrition. Most people who are able to eat well and exercise regularly for years and years without relapse do it because of the great rewards of good health — and not because of their constant fear of the grim reaper. The stick may be what first gets you moving, but the carrot will keep you rolling for the rest of the trip.

Towards that end, I have a few practical hints:

1) Don't worry about money. High quality food seems expensive, but in modern society even seemingly overpriced organic vegetables, fruits, and meats are really quite a bargain in the overall scheme of things. Same with supplements, nutraceuticals, and functional foods. Buy the best. Don't be driven by price. Surely there are other things less important than your health that you can give up if your budget is tight. Remember, if you save a single day in the hospital you will have justified years of seemingly exorbitant spending at the health food store.

2) Don't fret over the occasional cheat. Go ahead and have that slice of chocolate cheese cake after a special celebration at a fancy restaurant. You may be surprised to find that the temptation will diminish naturally over time. But even if it doesn't, a blast of poison now and then won't ruin your regimen – provided you are endowed with a huge supply of antioxidants, and that it doesn't occur too frequently..

3) Don't forget the nonfood portions of a healthful lifestyle. This, unavoidably, implies regular exercise. It can be as simple as a half-hour of vigorous walking every day. But you really do have to do it. I have one friend who can only activate his TV when he is moving on his stationary bicycle.

Other nonfood strategies include drinking enough water and allowing more time for sleep. These can also be vital elements in your overall health plan.

Good dental care – because of the links between infection and many degenerative diseases – is another nonfood strategy with implications for your entire body.

4) Use *behavior linking* to establish a routine. Choose a regular task that you do every day, and associate it with taking your supplements, or your morning exercise walk, or your afternoon barley powder cocktail, or flossing your teeth. For example, I always drink my barley cocktail every evening when I do my daily computer backup. After only a few weeks I found it difficult to make a backup without that cocktail glass on my desk!

5) Keep reading. Browse the nutrition book section of your favorite health food or book store, and subscribe to a health-oriented magazine or two. Search for topics that interest you on the internet. It's a jungle of conflicting information, but with a little patience you will find a clear path to the information and the inspiration that you need.

If you want a helpful reminder of how significant your lifestyle is when it comes to your health, and you appreciate some easy suggestions for maintaining that health, subscribe to my free daily nutrition hints. It will keep you up-to-date on how our medical community is finally validating all the pointers that the alternative nutrition educators have been recommending for years.

ONE LINE ONLINE DAILY NUTRITION HINT

My free Table Talk nutrition hint-of-the-day has been an overwhelming success. I email a free, one sentence daily Table Talk Nutrition Hint to anyone who wants it. (Note: The hints are sent via email only.)

The short hints offer the latest nutrition information reported in prestigious medical journals. Some days I summarize information gleaned from my global expeditions to other countries — nutrition findings I have accumulated through sources that are both personal and clinical.

Best of all, the hints serve as a daily reminder of how our lifestyle reflects our health and longevity. They suggest practical real-world ways to keep healthy and to improve compromised health.

The last ten hints are always available at the website (www.bettykamen.com), and include expanded information and source references.

To sign up for the free daily hints, just email to

betty@well.com

and write "hint" in the subject area.
No hype, no commercials, no cost.

ABOUT BETTY KAMEN

Years ago, on her popular radio program in New York City, Betty Kamen alerted her listeners to dozens of newly available supplements and treatments. Her program quickly developed into a center for disseminating innovative research and discoveries, featuring interviews with prominent alternative health care pioneers from around the world. Betty has written many cutting-edge health books, including the bestselling *Hormone Replacement Therapy, Yes or No? How to Make an Informed Decision.*

She received her MA in psychology in 1949, an MA in nutrition education in 1979, and her PhD in nutrition education in 1982. Betty taught at Hofstra University, developed a nutrition workshop at Stanford University Continuing Education Program for Doctors and Nurses, and served as nutrition consultant on the Committee of the Accrediting Council for Continuing Education and Training, Washington, DC.

A columnist for many health publications over the years, Betty has had hundreds of nutrition reports published. Articles written by or about Betty have appeared in the *New York Times, Chicago Tribune, San Francisco Progress, Prevention Magazine, Baltimore Sun,* and many other local and national publications. A full page photo of Betty and one of her grandchildren appeared in the March 1998 issue of *Time Magazine.*

But never mind all the credentials. Betty says her children describe her most aptly when they say, "Mom? She's just the oldest health nut in the country." To which Betty responds: "If you have to be the oldest anything, 'health nut' is not so bad."

ABOUT PAUL KAMEN

Paul Kamen is a naval architect with degrees from Webb Institute of Naval Architecture and the University of California at Berkeley. After his postgraduate degrees, he studied anthropology at the New School for Social Research in New York.

In addition to his technical consulting work, he writes a column for a monthly sailing magazine and chairs the Berkeley Waterfront Commission.

Paul helps out with some of his mother's more interesting research and writing projects. He is a lifelong consumer of nutraceuticals and functional foods, beginning with brewer's yeast at age two. (You might even say he started *in utero*; his mom ate lots of green vegetables and excellent food-type supplements during her pregnancy.)

While in college, he was arrested in a restaurant while driving back from a sailing competition for taking too many vitamins. He had an array of supplements on the table, and he was apprehended by the police who were out looking for students taking drugs. After narcotics detectives determined that the "pills" were in fact vitamins, he was released with an apology. In fact, the Stratford, Connecticut police precinct even paid for his dinner.

Paul lives with his wife Casilda and son Rocky in the hills above Berkeley, California, and races a small sailboat on San Francisco Bay.

Also From Betty Kamen

BOOKS

~ The Remarkable Healing Power of Velvet Antler
~ Hormone Replacement Therapy: Yes or No?
     How to Make an Informed Decision
~ Kamut
     An Ancient Food for a Healthy Future
~ Everything You Always Wanted to Know About
     Potassium But Were Too Tired to Ask
~ New Facts About Fiber
     How Fiber Supplements Can Enhance Your Health
~ The Chromium Connection
     Diet & Supplement Strategy for Blood Sugar Control
~ Startling New Facts About Osteoporosis
     Why Calcium Alone Does Not Prevent Bone Disease
~ Germanium
     A New Approach to Immunity
~ Siberian Ginseng
     Up-to-Date Research on the Fabled Tonic Herb
~ Sesame—The Superfood Seed
     How It Can Add Vitality to Your Life
~ Nutrition In Nursing—The New Approach
     A Handbook of Nursing Science
~ Osteoporosis
     What It Is, How to Prevent It, How to Stop It
~ In Pursuit of Youth
     Everyday Nutrition for Everyone Over 35
~ Kids Are What They Eat
     What Every Parent Needs to Know About Nutrition

~ Total Nutrition for Breast-Feeding Mothers

~ Total Nutrition During Pregnancy
     How To Be Sure You and Your Baby Are Eating the
     Right Stuff

Betty Kamen's Newest Book
on Female Sexuality
SHE'S GOTTA HAVE IT

Explores the reasons behind serious female sexuality problems, and offers simple self-help solutions. Frank and accurate, the style is light and easy to understand. Through it all, humor prevails.

TAPES

~ Table Talk Tapes: Lessons in Nutrition
   Six 1-hour Audio Cassette Tapes
      1. Supplements, 2. Food & Immunity, 3. Memory,
      4. Remedies, 5. Antioxidants (OPCs or Pycnogenol),
      6. Osteoporosis
~ Nutrition Breakthroughs
   Six 1-hour Audio Cassette Tapes
      1. Supplements, 2. Heart Health, 3. Scaling down,
      4. Immunity, 5. & 6. Common Problems
~ Individual Audio Tapes
      Locker Room Logic: For Men Only
      Things Your Mother Couldn't Tell You
      Hormonal Feedback
      Feminine and Afflicted
      Lactoferrin
             Helper Cells, Antioxidants, Immunity
      Cytolog
             Infopeptides and Cell Signaling
      Germanium
             Immunity, Alertness, Acuity

See www.bettykamen.com for details on all tapes, and for Betty Kamen's newsletters and special reports on new products.

REFERENCES

Chapter 1

1 *American Journal of Clinical Nutrition* 1999;70:307-308,412-419.

2 *Journal of Neuroscience* 1999 Sep15:19(18):8114-21.

3 Newsweek (United States), Dec 6 1999, 134(23) p91-2.

4 *American Journal of Respiratory Critical Care Medicine* 2000;161:1563-1566.

5 *Journal of Asthma* 2000;37:353-360.

6 World Alzheimer Congress 2000, Rotterdam, the Netherlands.

7 *Journal of the National Cancer Institute* 1999;91:605-613.

8 *European Journal of Cancer* 2000;36:636-646.

9 *Preventive Medicine* 1999;28:333-339.

10 *American Journal of Clinical Nutrition* 1999;70(4):517-24.

11 *Journal of Agriculture and Food Chemistry* 2002 May 22;50(11):3346-50.

12 *Gastroenterology* 2000;118:1233-1257.

13 *American Journal of Clinical Nutrition* 2000;71(2):575-82.

14 Nahrung 1997 Apr;41(2):68-74.

15 *Journal of Clinical Epidemiology* 1999 Apr;52(4):329-35.

16 *American Journal of Clinical Nutrition* July 1999; 70(1): 85-90.

17 *Diseases of the Colon and Rectum* 2000 Oct;43(10):1412-8.

18 *Cancer Control: Journal of the Moffitt Cancer Center* 2000;7(3):288-296, 2000.

19 *Thorax* 1999;54:1021-1026.

20 *Journal of the National Cancer Institute* 2000; 92(22):1812-1823

21 *American Journal of Clinical Nutrition,* 1999; 69:727-36.

22 *Nature* 1999;401:343-344.

23 *Journal of the National Cancer Institute* 2000;92:61-68.

24 *American Journal of Clinical Nutrition* 1999 Dec;70(6):1077-82.

25 CBS Health Watch, Sep 26, 2000.

26 *Lancet* 1998;351:687.

27 *American Journal of Clinical Nutrition* 72;2000:929-36.

28 *Appetite* 2000 Dec;35(3):251-262.

29 Ralph Waldo Emerson, *Essays,*" Nature" (Second Series, 1844).

30 *American Journal of Clinical Nutrition* 2000;72(5):1214-1222.

31 *New England Journal of Medicine* 1997;336(22):1569-1574.

32 *American Journal of Clinical Nutrition* 2002;76 1-2.

33 *Annals of Allergy Asthma Immunology* 1998;81:347-351.

34 *Lancet*, Dec 22/29, 1984, "Headed in the Wrong Direction," D Burkitt, p 1475.

CHAPTER 2

1 Public Interest Research Groups, May 23, 2002.

2 S Gursche, *Encyclopedia of Natural Healing* (Burnaby, Canada: Alive Books, 1998) 121-122.

3 *Nutrition Reviews* 1999, in press.

4 S Kanaan. Report presented at FASEB, April 19, 1999.

5 *Journal of the American Medical Association* 1999;282:1233-1239.

6 *European Journal of Epidemiology* Jul 1999;15(6):507-515.

7 *Prostaglandins, Leukotrines, and Essential Fatty Acids* 1999:60(5-6):421-429.

8 *Przeglad Lekarski* [Polish] 1999;56(3):211-215.

9 Reuters Medical News Service, Westport, Mar 29, 2002..

10 *American Journal of Clinical Nutrition* 2000;72(2):476-483.

11 *Annals of the Review of Public Health* 1998;19:73-99.

12 *Journal of the American Medical Association* 1996;275:699-703.

13 *Journal of Agricultural Research* Feb 1999.

14 *Epidemiology* 1999;10:679-684.
15 *American Journal of Clinical Nutrition* Oct 1999;70(4):431-432.
16 *Nature* 2000;405:902-904.
17 *Carcinogenesis* 1999;20(12):2267-2272.
18 *New England Journal of Medicine* 2000;342:154-160.
19 *Nutrition Reviews* 1998;56:S49.
20 *Nutrition* 1989;297(5).
21 *Journal of the Nutrition Institute* 1980;65(4):671-674.
22 Reuters Medical Report, Nov 5, 1999.
23 HF DeLuca, *Vitamin D: Metabolism and Function* (NY: Springer-Verlag, 1970).
24 Canadian Cardiovascular Congress, 2000, Montreal.
25 *Lancet*, Dec 22/29, 1984:1475.

CHAPTER 3
1 *British Medical Journal* 2000;321:93-96 (8 July)
2 *Immunology Today* 1999 Mar;20(3):108-10.
3 *Diabetes Metabolism Review* 1997 Sep;13(3):127-38.
4 British Medical Journal, op cit.
5 *Circulation* 1999 Apr 13;99(14):1885-91.
6 *Clinical Cardiology* 1999 Apr;22(4):292-6.
7 *Journal of Internal Medicine* 1999 Feb;245(2):199-203.
8 *Gut Reactions* (Broadway Books, NY), p 51.
9 Fertil Steril 2001;76:223-231.
10 P154 XXX Get full ref Imm book
11 Mutation research 1989;225:131-6.
12 *Nutrition Modulation Of The Immune Response* (Marcel Dekker, NY,
          1993).
13 FASEB Meeting, SF 1998.
14 *Archives of Internal Physiology* 1986;94:529-34.
15 *Journal of Lipid Research* 1979;20:639-45.
16 *Modern Nutrition in Health and Disease,* 8th ed (Lea and Febiger,
          Philadelphia 1994).
17 *Nutrition and Immunity: Principles & Pracitce,* ed ME Gershin (NJ: Humana Press,
          Inc, 2000), p 186.
18 Op cit, p 190
19 *American Journal of Clinical Nutrition* 1997;66:464-72.
20 *American Journal of Gastroenterology* 2001;96:1751-1757.
21 "Infectious Diseases Take Center Stage." Feb 18, 1999,
          Medical Tribune.
22 *Journal of Clinical Investigation* 2001;108:311-318.
23 *American Journal of Indian Medicie* Med 2001;40:199-210.
24 *Journal of Nutrition.* 2001;131:2798S-2804S.
25 *Ibid.*
26 *Human Reproduction* 2001;16:2333-2337.
27 Interscience Conference on Antimicrobial Agents and Chemotherapy,
          Chicago, 2001.
28 Thorax 2001;56:290-295,
29 *British Medical Journal* 2000;321:93-96 (8 July).
30 *Lancet* 2001;357:858.
31 *American Journal of Gastroenterology* 2001;96:773-775.
32 *Antimicrobial Agents* 2001;45:1721-1729.

Chapter 4

1 *Australian Family Physician* 1994;23(7):1297-301,1305.

2 *Canadian Respiratory Journal* 2000 Nov-Dec;7(6):476-80.

3 *Turkish Journal of Pediatrics* 2000 Jan-Mar;42(1):17-21.

4 Pol Merkuriusz Lek 2001 Nov;11(65):385-8

5 *Thorax* Feb 1997;52(2):166-170.

6 *American Journal of Respiratory and Critical Care* 1994;150:S77-9.

7 *Terapevticheskii Arkhiv* 1994;66(3):32-34.

8 *Journal of Biological Chemistry* 2002 Jun 21;277(25):22814-21

9 Pneumonol Alergol Pol 2001;69(9-10):553-63

10 *Polish Merkuriusz Lek* 2001 Nov;11(65):385-8

11 Journal of Nutritional Biochemistry 2001 Mar;12(3):144-152.

12 *Journal of the American College of Nutrition* 1999 Oct;18(5):451-61.

13 *Free Radical Biology Medicine* Apr 1999, 26(7-8) p892-904.

14 *Free Radical Research* 1997 Jul;27(1).

15 *Atherosclerosis* 2002 Apr;161(2):307-16.

16 *Circulation* 1994 Dec;90(6):3118-9.

17 *Cardiovasc Research* 2002 Jun;54(3):503-15.

18 *Chemical Biology* 1999 Jun;6(6):R157-66.

19 *Clinical Science* (London) 2001 Dec;101(6):593-9.

20 *British Journal of Nutrition* 2001 Mar;85(3):251-69.

21 *Clinical Chim Acta* 1999 Jun 15;284(1):45-58.

22 *Vestnik Dermatologii*, 1990.

23 *Cancer Epidemiology Biomarkers Preview* 2002 Jan;11(1):7-13.

24 *Journal of the American Medical Association* July 26, 2002;287(24):3223-
        3237,3261=3263.

25 *Clinical Biochemistry* 2000 Jun;33(4):279-84.

26 *Disease Markers* 1999 Dec;15(4):283-91.

27 Kellman R. *Gut Reactions* (New York: Broadway Books, 2002), p 251.

28 *Prostaglandins Leukotrioneols and Essential Fatty Acids* 2001 Sep;65(3):165-71.

29 *Journal of Nutrition* 2002 Jan;132(1):121-4.

30 *Nutrition and Cancer* 1999;34(1):100-10.

31 *Japanese Journal of Cancer and Chemotherapy*, 1993.

32 *American Journal of Medicine*, 1994.

33 *Diseases of the Colon and Rectum*, March 1993.

34 *Experimenta Supplement*, from Basel, 1992.

35 *Nutrition* 2001 Oct;17(10):828-34.

CHAPTER 5

1 B Jensen, *Chlorella: Gem of the Orient* (Escondido, CA: Bernard Jensen Intl., 1987),
        p 24.

2 *Journal of the American Academy of Dermatology* Dec 1997;37(6):942-947.

3 *Nutrition, Metabolism and Cardiovascular Diseases* Aug 2001;11(4 Suppl):74-77.

4 *Annals of Tropical Pediatrics* Sep 2000;20(3):217-221.

5 *Cancer* March 2002;94:1867-1875.

6 *Australian and New Zealand Journal of Public Health* Apr 2002;26(2):108-115.

7 *Frontiers in Bioscience* Apr 1, 2002;7:d784-792.

8 RL Seibold, *Cereal Grass: What's In It For You!* (Lawrence, Kansas: Wilderness
        Community Education Foundation, 1990), p 13.

9 *Critical Reviews in Food Science and Nutrition* 1980;13(4):353-385.

10 Yoshihide. Hagiwara, M.D., *Green Barley Essence: The Ideal Fast Food* (New
        Canaan, CT: Keats Publishing, 1985), pp 69-70.

11 *Mutation Research* Oct 18 2001;497(1-2):139-145.

12 *Carcinogenesis* 1991;12(5):939-942.

13 *Teratogens, Carcinogens, and Mutagens* 1994;14(2):75-81.

CHAPTER 6

1 *Cancer Letters* Jan 25, 2002;175(2):129-139.
2. EM Haas, *Staying Healthy With Nutrition: The Complete Guide to Diet and Nutritional Medicine*. (Berkeley, CA: Celestial Arts, 1992), 272,728.
3 *Japanese Heart Journal* Jan 2002;43(1):25-34.
4 *Hepato-gastroenterology* Jul-Aug 2001;48(40):1102-1105.
5 *Movement Disorders* Jul 2001;16(4):705-707.
6 *Cochrane Database Systematic Review* 2001;(1):CD001968.
7 *Science* Sep 1, 2000;289(5484):1567-1569.
8 *Acta Biochimica Polonica* 1999;46(2):249-253.
9 *Biochemical and Biophysical Research Communications*, 2000;270(3):714-716.
10 *Lancet* Feb 19, 2000;355(9204):624.
11 *Research in Experimental Medicine* (Berlin) Dec 1999;199(3):167-176.
12 *Journal of Investigative Dermatology* Nov 1999;113(5):843-847.
13 *Journal of Nutrition* 1993;123:803-810.
14 *Annals of Clinical Biochemistry* 1978;15:293-296.
15 *Toxicology and Applied Pharmacology* March 1, 2002;179(2):65-73.
16. HA Guthrie, *Introductory Nutrition*. (St. Louis, MI: CV Mosby Co., 1983).
17 *Journal of the National Cancer Institute* 1989;81:21.
18 *Journal of Nutrition* Jun 2002;132(6):1368-1375.
19 *Photochemistry and Photobiology* May 2002;75(5):503-506.
20 *Phytochemical Analysis: PCA* Mar-Apr 2001;12(2):138-143.
21 *Journal of Nutrition* Mar 2002;132(3):540S-542S.
22 *Journal of Nutrition* Dec 2001;131(12):3303-3306.
23 *Journal of Nutrition* Dec 1999;129(12):2162-2169.
24 *Journal of Chromatography. A* Jul 27, 2001;924(1-2):519-522.
25 *International Journal of Cancer* Apr 15, 2001;92(2):298-302.
26 *American Journal of Clinical Nutrition* May 2001;73(5):941-948.
27 *International Journal of Cancer* Apr 15, 2001;92(2):298-302.
28 *AIDS* Apr 12, 2002;16(6):939-941.
29 B Kamen, P Kamen, *The Remarkable Healing Power of Velvet Antler* (Nutrition Encounter, Novato,CA, 1999).
30 *Nuclear Medicine Communications* Jan 2002;23(1):53-59.
31. *Journal of Agriculture and Food Chemistry* Dec 2001;49(12):6033-6038.
32 *American Journal of Clinical Nutrition* Aug 2001;74(2):227-232.
33 *Cancer Research* Jan 1, 2001;61(1):118-125.
34 *Archives of Internal Medicine* 1999;10/11
35 *European Journal of Clinical Nutrition* Feb 2001;55(2):76-81.
36. S Levine, PM. Kidd, *Antioxidation Adaptation: Its Role in Free Radical Pathology*. (San Leandro, CA: Allergy Research Group, 1986), p 294.
37 *Journal of Ophthalmic Nursing Technology* 1993;12(5):217-224.
38 P Quillin, *Healing Nutrients: The People's Guide to Using Common Nutrients That Will Help You Feel Better Than You Ever Thought Possible* (NY: M Evans & Co, Inc, 1990), p 264.
39 *Age and Ageing* May 2001;30(3):23.
40 *Journal of Dental Research* 1963;42:233-244
41 *American Journal of Clinical Nutrition* 2000;75(1):92-98.
42 *American Journal of Clinical Nutrition* 1991;53:1087-1101.
43 *Journal of the American Medical Association* 2002;287:47-54.
44 *Journal of Nutrition* 2002;132:197-203.
45 *Anticancer Research* 2000 May-Jun;20(3B):2245-8.
46 *Journal of Neurochemistry* 1997 Nov;69(5):2005-10.

47 *Neurochemistry International* 2002 May;40(6):493-504.

48. Personal communication, M Rosenbaum, MD.

49 *American Journal of Clinical Nutrition* Aug 2000;72(2 Suppl):598S-606S.

50. *International Journal of Epidemiology*.

51 *Preventive Medicine* Jan 1993.

52 *Cancer*

53 *Anticancer Research* Sep 1990.

54 *Voprosy Onkologii* 1992;38:141.

55 *Biological Chemistry* Mar-Apr 2002;383(3-4):671-681.

56. *Environmental Health Perspectives* 2001;109:1007-1009.

57 B Kamen, *She's Gotta Have It* (Nutrition Encounter: Novato, CA, 2002).

58 42nd annual conference on Cardiovascular Disease and Epidemiology Prevention, April 2002, Honolulu, Hawaii.

59 *Arthritis and Rheumatism* Feb 2002;46(2):522-532.

60 *Proceedings of the National Academy of Sciences* 2002;99:7408-7413.

61 *Annals of New York Academy of Sciences* Dec 2001;952:145-152.

62 *Age and Ageing* May 2001;30(3):23.

63 *Journal of the American Medical Association* 2002;287:3223-3237,3261-3263.

64 *Archives of Neurology* 2002;59:1125-1132.

65 R Moore, G Webb, *The K Factor: Reversing and Preventing High Blood Pressure Without Drugs*. (NY: MacMillan, 1986), p 215.

66 J Scala, *The High Blood Pressure Relief Diet*. (NY: Penguin, 1990), p 52.

67 *British Medical Journal* (Clinical Research ed) April 7, 2001;322:811-812.

68 *Nutrition Reviews* 1996;54:295-317.

69. R Rhoades, R Pflanzer, *Human Physiology* (NY: Harcourt Brace Jovanovich, 1992), p 218.

70. A Cichoke, *Living Naturally, Let's Live*.

CHAPTER 7

1 *American Journal of Clinical Nutrition* 2002;76:259.

2 *Lancet* 1998:352(SIV):2.

3 *Postgraduate Medicine* Mar 1999;105(3):173-181.

4 *Radiation Research* Sep 2000;154(3):261-267.

5 *Carcinogenesis* Jun 1999;20(6):1005-1009.

6 *Digestive Diseases and Sciences* Sep 1998;43(9):2055-2060.

7 *Bioscience, Biotechnology and Biochemistry* Apr 2001;65(4):774-780.

8 *Journal of Nutritional Science and Vitaminology* (Tokyo) Dec 2001;47(6):367-372.

9 *Journal of Nutrition* 2001;131(3s):1010S-1015S.

10 Ibid:1075S-1079S.

11 Ibid:1071S-1074S.

12 Ibid:1020S-1026S.

13 Ibid:1016S-1019S.

14 Ibid:1093S-1095S.

15 Ibid:977S-979S.

16 *Journal of Ethnopharmacology* Oct 2000;72(3):345-393.

17 *European Journal of Pharmacology* Feb 2, 2002;436(3):151-158.

18 B Kamen, *Hormone Replacement Therapy, Yes or No?: How to Make an Informed Decision*. (Novato, CA: Nutrition Encounter, 2002), p 236.

19 *Alternative Medicine Review* Feb 2000;5(1):4-27.

20 *Mutation Research* Sep 20, 2001;496(1-2):5-13.

21 *Journal of Endocrinology* May 1998;157(2):259-266.

22 *Caries Research* Jan-Feb 2000;34(1):94-98.

23 *Journal of Agriculture and Food Chemistry* Nov 2001;49(11):5461-5467.

24 *Life Sciences* 1997;60(10):763-771.

25 *Food and Chemical Toxicology* Apr 1998;36(4):315-320.
26 B Kamen, P Kamen *The Remarkable Healing Power of Velvet Antler*. (Novato, CA: Nutrition Encounter, 1999), p 17.
27 *American Journal of Clinical Nutrition* Jun 2002;75(6):1084-1092.
28. *Journal of the American College of Nutrition* Oct 2000;19(5 Suppl):499S-506S.
29 *Applied Microbiology and Biotechnology* Oct 2001;57(3):282-286.
30 *Journal of the Pakistan Medical Association* Jun 2000;50(6):204-207.
31 *Life Sciences* Feb 15, 2002;70(13):1509-1518.
32 *Advances in Experimental Medicine and Biology* 2001;492:69-81.
33 *Lancet* 2002;359:2003-2004.
34 *American Journal of Clinical Nutrition* 1999;70.
35 *BMJ* 1999;319:815-819.
36. *Journal of the National Cancer Institute* 1999;91:1765-1772.
37. *Indian Pediatrics* 2001;38:381-384.
38. Annual meeting of the American Academy of Pediatricians, 2001, San Francisco.
39 *Journal of Nutrition* Mar 1997;127(3):436-443.
40 *American Journal of Clinical Nutrition* May 2002;75(5):914-921.
41 *Archives of Diseases in Childhood* 2002;86:400-402.
42 *Lancet* 2002;360:187-195.
43 *Gut* Nov 1998;43(5):699-704.
44 *Critical Review of Food Science and Nutrition* Aug 1998;38(6):421-464.
45 *South African Medical Journal* Apr 14, 1979;55(16):631-632.
46 Society of Behavioral Medicine, March 2000, San Diego, CA.
47 *Comparative Biochemistry and Physiology. Part C: Pharmacology, Toxicology, & Endocrinology* Jan 1997;116(1):39-45.
48 *Mutation Research* Feb 19, 1996;350(1):153-161.
49 *Neuroscience Letters* Aug 18, 1995;196(1-2):85-88.
50 *Cancer Letters* Feb 28, 1994;77(1):33-38.
51 *Journal of Nutrition* May 2002;132(5):1062S-1101S.
52 *Current Opinion in Clinical Nutrition and Metabolic Care* Nov 1999;2(6):481-484.
53 *Reproduction, Nutrition, Development* Sep-Dec 1999;39(5-6):563-588.

CHAPTER 8
1 *Journal of Renal Nutrition* Apr 2002;12(2):76-86.
2 *International Journal of Antimicrobial Agents* Dec 2000;16(4):531-536.
3 Ibid:531-536.
4 *European Journal of Pediatrics* Oct 2001;160(10):592-594.
5 *Current Opinion in Lipidology* Feb 1998;9(1):7-10.
6 *Journal of Renal Nutrition* Apr 2002;12(2):76-86.
7 *American Journal of Health-System Pharmacy* Jun 15, 2001;58(12):1101-1109.
8 *Journal of Pediatric Gastroenterology and Nutrition* Oct 2001;33(S2):S17-S25.
9 *Acta Medica Croatica* 1999;53(1):23-28.
10 Bibek Ray, Mark Daeschel, *Food Biopreservatives of Microbial Origin*. (Boca Raton, FL: CRC Press, 1992), 17-21.
11 *American Journal of Clinical Nutrition* Feb 2001;73(2 Suppl):430S-436S.
12 *Current Opinion in Microbiology* Jun 2000;3(3):276-282.
13 *Gynecology and Obstetrics Investigations* 1986;21:19-25.
14 *Journal of Nutrition* Jun 2002;132(6):1173-1175.
15 *Letters in Applied Microbiology* Dec 1998;27(6):345-348.
16 *Journal of Food Protection* Sep 2001;64(9):1439-1441.
17 *Antonie Van Leeuwenhoek* Jul-Nov 1999;76(1-4):293-315.
18 *Journal of Renal Nutrition* Apr 2002;12(2):76-86.
19 *Journal of Nutrition* Jul 1999;129(7 Suppl):1478S-1482S.
20 *American Journal of Clinical Nutrition* Feb 2001;73(2 Suppl):459S-464S.

21 *Nutrition* Jan 1997;127(1):130-136.

22 *British Journal of Nutrition* Oct 1998;80(4):S209-S212.

23 *Journal of the American Dietetic Association* 1992;92(6):698-704,707.

24 *Magnesium Research* 1992;5(1):15-21.

25 *Nutrition and Cancer* 1992;17(2):139-151.

26 S Gursche, *Encyclopedia of Natural Healing*. (Burnaby, Canada: Alive Books, 1997), p 218.

Chapter 9

1 Interview with Loren Cordain, PhD, by Robert Crayhon, MS;
http://www.lifeservices.com/cordain.htm
Loren Cordain, PhD, can be contacted at:
Professor, Department of Exercise & Sports Science
Colorado State University
Fort Collins, Colorado 80523 USA

2 The origins of agriculture – a biological perspective and a new hypothesis, by Greg Wadley & Angus Martin, Department of Zoology, University of Melbourne. Published in Australian Biologist 6: 96 – 105, June 1993
http://www.edfac.unimelb.edu.au/EPM/papers/GW_paper.html

INDEX

A

Acid/alkaline balance 139,142,146
Acne 129
Additives 27
Aging 15,57,68,88,89
Allergies 10,15,41,27
Alpha carotene 91,92
Alpha carotenoids 121
Alpha lipoic acid 121
Alzheimer's disease 15,64,98,106
Anabolic 83
Anemia 42,84
Anthocyanins 91
Antibiotic 51,134
Antibodies 45-47
Antioxidants 15,37,52-68,72,103,104
Anxiety 100
Aphrodisiacs 124
Apples 37,75
Arginine/lysine ratio 131
Aristotle 54
Arthritis 15,41,63,94,123
Aspirin 51,99
Asthma 15,50,61,89
Atherosclerosis 57
Athletes 83
Autoimmunity 41-43,50

B

B cells 45
B vitamins 99,115,121
Bad breath 136
Barley 9,11
Barley food 114
Barley green facts 146
Barley grass and alkalinity 146
Barley, as green sprouts 12-13
Beets, crystallized 114
Beta-carotene 22,49,58,65,91,92

BHT 59
Biological memory 41
Blood 79,109
Blood pressure 128
Bologna 53,136
Bread 148
Breast milk 128
Brewer's yeast 33,115
Bronchial spasms 84
Brown rice 121
Burkitt, MD, Denis 142

C

Caffeine 130
Calcium 39,101,108,109
Cancer 42,47,57.58.65,71,89,100,118
Cancer, bladder 15
Cancer, breast 15,71,102,126,128
Cancer, colon 16,66,71
Cancer, digestive tract 16
Cancer, endometriosis 17
Cancer, ovarian 71
Cancer, prostate 17
Candida 136
Cardiovascular disease 16,42,84
Carotene 60,77,90,93
Carotenoids 37,49,90,93,121
Carpal tunnel syndrome 100
Catabolic 83
Cataracts 16,57,67
Catechins 69,94-95
Celiac disease 128
Chickenpox 41,70-85,90,92
Chlorine 28
Chlorophyll 70-85
Chlorophyll molecule 80
Cholesterol 16,100,118,136
Chondroitin sulfate 123
Chromosomes 9
Co Q10 121
Coble, MD, Yank 36
Collagen 94
Colostrum 116

Cordain, PhD, Loren 149
Coronary heart disease 62,130
Corsello, Serafina 3
Crohn's disease 104
Cutter, MD, Richard 110
D
Deer 123
Dehydration 74,75
Dementia 64
Detoxification 136
DHA 125
Diabetes 16,42,50,66
Diarrhea 137
Dietary Guidelines 20,69,86
Diverticulosis 16
DNA 65,69,85,103,110
Drugs 60
E
Eczema 63,64,129
Eggs 73,125
Elk 123
Endometriosis 43
Enzymes
  32,58,74,88,90,108,110,112
Eosinophils 51
Essential fatty acids 125,126
Estrogen 101
Exercise 88,106
Exorphin 150
F
Fermented foods 137,139
Fertility 124
Fever 44
Fiber 142-145
Fiber Quiz 143-144
Finland 63
Fish 29
Flavonoids 66,86,91
Flax seed 125-127,131
Flouride 23
Folic acid 100
France 63
Free radical 56-58,63,88
Fried foods 88

Functional foods 31,33,34
Functional foods, list 113
G
Gamma oryzenol 120
Garbage study 76
Garlic 127-128,131
Garlic, aged 117
Genetically modified foods 27
Genistein 38
Gingivitis 90
Ginseng, Korean 118
Ginseng, Siberian 118
Ginter, MD, Emil 62
Glucosamine sulfate 123
Glucose 78
Glutathione peroxidase
Grapeseed oil 131
Grave's disease 42
Growth factors 116
H
H pylori 50
Hagiwara,MD, Yoshide 79
Hashioto's thyroiditis disease 42
Healthful foods 68
Heart disease 63,130
Heart flutters 38
Heber, MD, David 14
Hemoglobin 79,80,109
Hemoglobin molecule 80
Hepatitis C 50
Hip fracture 70,99
Homocysteine 101,195
Hot dogs 19,20,53,136
Hypertension 130
I
Immunity 22,24,40-51,119
Immunity and green leaf barley 48
Immunoglobulins 124
India 122
Infection 41,47,50
Infertility 50
Inflammation 41,44,90,105
Inflammatory bowel disease 50

Insoluble fiber 144
Insulin 118
Iron 38,49,79,80,109,129,142
Ischemia 57,89,95
J
Japan 118,147
Jaundice 71
Jointing stage 73
K
Kandel, MD, Herb 118
L
Lactic acid bacteria 138-149
Lactobacillus 138
Lactose intolerance 138
Laser eye surgery 67
LDL cholesterol 62,66
Leaf 84
Lettuce 80,82
Leukemia 50
Linoleic acid 126
Linolenic acid 126
Lipase 120
Lung cancer 17,66
Lung disease 64,89
Lung function 17
Lupus 43
Lutein 91
Lycopene 91
Lysine/arginine ratio 131
M
Macrophage 44,61
Macular degeneration 66,93
Magnesium 79,80,84,126
Martin, Angus 150
Melanoma 72,102,103
Memory cells 45
Menopausal symptoms 84
Mercury 29
Milk, human 128
Minerals 106
Mon0cytes 51
Multiple sclerosis 42,51
Multivitamins 39
Mumps 41

Muscle cramping 84
Mushroom, extracts 118
Mushrooms 129
Myasthenia gravis 42
Myocardial damage 42
N
Neolithic lifestyle 26
Netherlands 95
Neutrophils 44,51
Niacin 100
Nitrites 53
Nucleic acids 85
Nutraceuticals 112-133
O
Oil 125-126
Oligosaccharides 141-142
Omega 3 126,130
Omega 6 130
Organ meats 29
Osteoporosis 17,63,108
Ott,MD, John 71
Oxidants 55
Oxidation 49,54-55,57
Oxidative stress 66
Oxide radicals 89
Oxygen 78,110
P
Paleolithic diet 30-31,149
Palm oil 92
Pancreatic cancer 66
Parkinson's disease 57.89,95
Pasteurization 109
Pathogens 43,45,46,51
Pepperoni pizza 19
Peptic ulcers 50
Peroxides 88
Pest resistance 10
Pesticides 80
pH 139,142
Phagocytes 51,110
Phosphorous 101
Photosynthesis 78,89,104
Phytochemicals 87
Phytosterols 121

Pigments 15,77.91
Plaque 62
Platelet aggregation 62
PMS 100
Pollution 84
Polyphenols 60,121
Porphyrin ring 79
Potassium 106
Prebiotic 134,140-142
Probiotic 134-149
Progesterone 136
Prooxidant 38
Prostate cancer 91,102,106
Proteoglycens 94
Psychiatric disorders 50
Pus 46
Q
Quercitin 65,77
R
Respiration 78
Retina 91
Rheumatoid arthritis 17,57,63,89
Riboflavin 100,101
Rice bran, stabilized 120
Rickets 70
Rooibos tea 129
Ryokko Aojiru 147
S
Sauerkraut 34
Sclerosis 90
Sex hormones 57
Sexual function 105,123
Shizen green 147
SIDS 128
Skin cancer 72,102,103
Smoking 64,105
SOD 58,65,87-90,110,121,129
Sodium 106
Soluble fiber 144
South Africa 130
Spinach 36
Sprouts 32,34,73,104
Steroids 83
Streptococcal infection 50

Stress 57
Stroke 17,59,78,79,01,102,104
T
T cells 45
Table Talk Hints 153
Tannin 129
Thiamine 100
Thymus 51
Thyroid disease 42
T-lymphocytes 51
Tocopherols 120
Tuberculosis 51
Tumor 47
U
Ultraviolet radiation 71,101,102
Urinary tract infections 136
V
Vascular diseases 66
Vegetable oils 82
Velvet antler 123
Viagra 123
Virus 56
Vitamin B1 100,101
Vitamin B12 100,101
Vitamin B2 100,101
Vitamin B3 100
Vitamin B6 99,100,101
Vitamin A 34,38,90,92,96-99
Vitamin C 34,37,58,93,96,97
Vitamin D 39,70,101-104,126
Vitamin E 38,49,60,98,105
Vitamins 96-106
W
Walnuts 16,130-131
Wheat 7-11
White blood cells 51
Williams, Roger 23
Winter grasses 72
Wrinkles 57
X
Xenobiotic 59
Z
Zeaxanthin 91
Zinc 98,110-111